THE
BLUEPRINT
FOR BACK PAIN
RELIEF

THE
BLUEPRINT
FOR BACK PAIN
RELIEF

THE ESSENTIAL GUIDE TO
NON-SURGICAL
SOLUTIONS

BRADFORD T. BUTLER, DC

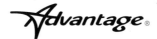

Published by Advantage, Charleston, South Carolina.
Member of Advantage Media Group.

ADVANTAGE is a registered trademark, and the Advantage colophon is a trademark of Advantage Media Group, Inc.

Printed in the United States of America.

10 9 8 7 6 5 4 3 2 1

ISBN: 978-1-59932-902-4
LCCN: 2018938205

Cover and layout design by George Stevens.

This publication is designed to provide accurate and authoritative information in regard to the subject matter covered. It is sold with the understanding that the publisher is not engaged in rendering legal, accounting, or other professional services. If legal advice or other expert assistance is required, the services of a competent professional person should be sought.

 Advantage Media Group is proud to be a part of the Tree Neutral® program. Tree Neutral offsets the number of trees consumed in the production and printing of this book by taking proactive steps such as planting trees in direct proportion to the number of trees used to print books. To learn more about Tree Neutral, please visit **www.treeneutral.com**.

Advantage Media Group is a publisher of business, self-improvement, and professional development books and online learning. We help entrepreneurs, business leaders, and professionals share their Stories, Passion, and Knowledge to help others Learn & Grow. Do you have a manuscript or book idea that you would like us to consider for publishing? Please visit **advantagefamily.com** or call **1.866.775.1696**.

To my wife, Kim, and my four incredible children,
Zack, Katie, Andrew, and Kelsie.

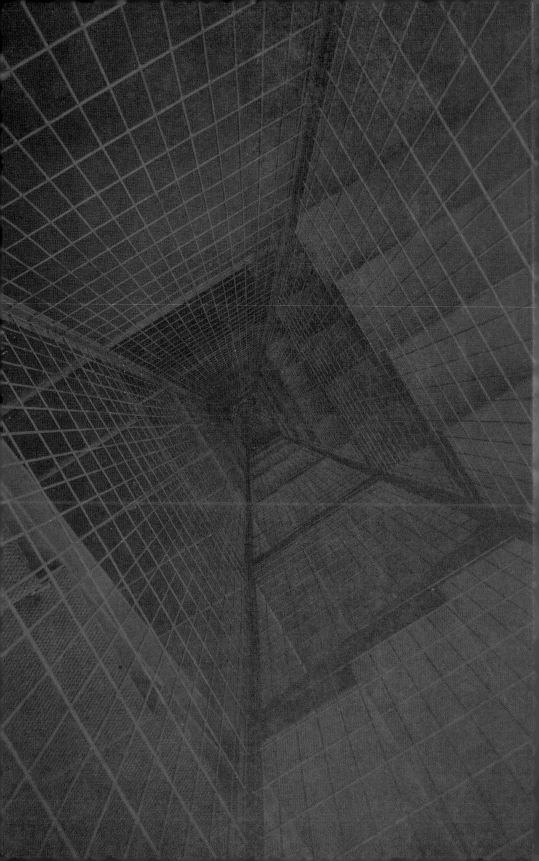

ABOUT THE AUTHOR

Bradford Butler, DC, graduated cum laude in 1995 with a doctor of chiropractic degree from New York Chiropractic College. He was named "One of America's Top Chiropractors" by Consumer Research Council of America, was awarded "NJ Top Doctor" eight years in a row by NJTopDocs.com and is a noted contributor to two *New York Times* best-selling books. He is a sought-after speaker inside and outside the chiropractic profession for Fortune 500 companies, international corporations, and schools and universities.

As owner and clinic director of Oakland Spine & Physical Therapy, Dr. Butler leads a team whose goal is to help people live longer, healthier, happier, and pain-free lives. Together, they are on a mission to serve patients across the United States by having Oakland Spine locations in every state, making patient-centric care accessible to everyone.

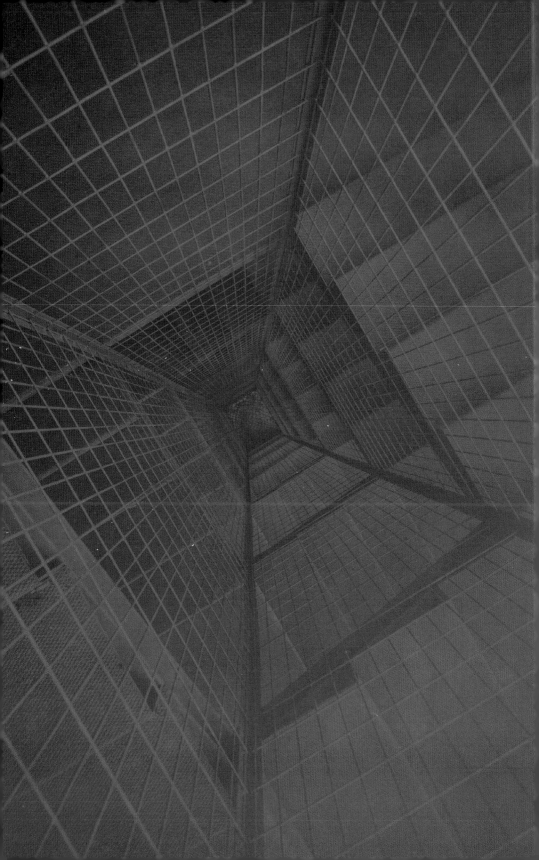

TABLE OF CONTENTS

THERE IS A BETTER WAY

What if everything you thought you knew about treating your back pain was wrong? What if the system for back pain was rigged against bringing you relief? What if the doctor you thought you could trust to get you the right information wasn't doing so—would you even want to know? Is it even possible for you to get the answers you need?

With billions of dollars being spent every year marketing solutions for back pain, and even more being spent on treatments, shouldn't you be feeling better by now? Shouldn't you have some relief for your chronic pain?

That's the purpose of this book. I want to "right the ship" for readers. I want to show you how the system for relieving back pain as you know it is upside down. And I want to let you in on a little secret I discovered more than ten years ago—a secret that is just now starting to be revealed by the scientific community.

In fact, my hope is that before you even finish reading this book, you'll already have begun altering your decision-making process.

You'll already be starting to see how to feel better and how to relieve your pain "the right way."

I'm going to share with you what twenty years of relentless pursuit of quality of life for my patients has revealed. I'm going to share with you how my team and I at Oakland Spine & Physical Therapy have successfully treated tens of thousands of patients. Without drugs or surgery, we've helped these patients recover from back and neck pain ranging from acute episodes to conditions so chronic and severe that the patient was bound to a wheelchair or walker—but can now walk again.

My dedication to relieving others of pain started with my own story back in eighth grade when my mom took me to a chiropractor—not for a back problem but for a sprained ankle. That visit to the chiropractor only came about after a chance encounter between my mom and her friend at the supermarket, who referred my mom. I had sprained my ankle during a summertime invitational basketball camp in the Poconos. After returning home and being unable to see the sports medicine doctor my family had used for years, my mom and I (on crutches) set off to run some errands. That's when we encountered my mom's friend, who upon hearing about our situation said, "Why don't you take him to my chiropractor?" The chiropractor was able to get me in that day and during his exam, he also looked at my lower back and pelvis. "If those

> **MY DEDICATION TO RELIEVING OTHERS OF PAIN STARTED WITH MY OWN STORY BACK IN EIGHTH GRADE WHEN MY MOM TOOK ME TO A CHIROPRACTOR— NOT FOR A BACK PROBLEM BUT FOR A SPRAINED ANKLE.**

aren't properly aligned, it can predispose him to more ankle injuries," he explained.

His examination then found problems all along my spine, which prompted him to ask whether I had a lot of other ailments. Sure enough, as a child, I was sick quite often with allergies and other illnesses. Although I was always loading up on over-the-counter medications and being prescribed antibiotics for this and that, I still ended up with a couple of bouts of bronchitis every year.

It turned out that all my problems stemmed from a weak immune system. Until the chiropractor explained how that was happening, no one had ever addressed a weak immune system as the source of my problems. I was amazed a "bone doctor" would have a clue about anything other than what I thought was his area of expertise. He explained to my mom that the reason I was sick all the time was because the nerves exiting my spine in the upper neck, upper back, and mid-back controlled the function of my lungs and other organs along with my immune system, and they needed treatment. In medicine, "health" is defined as "100 percent function"—it's not about how you feel, it's about how well your systems are functioning. The chiropractor explained that a lot of people get sick not because of an invasion of germs, but because the immune system can't keep those germs in check.

He explained that with regular treatment, there was a good chance he could help my ankle and strengthen my overall immune system. I walked out of that appointment filled with hope that my days of pills and shots were over. After undergoing his treatments, not only did my allergies and bronchitis disappear forever, but I decided that I wanted to do the same thing for other people as he had done for me.

That's how my practice got started. It all began with that encounter when I was in the eighth grade. Since becoming a chiropractor myself, I've devoted my career to treating and teaching people that there is nothing better for successfully treating back pain, no matter how severe. But I've also learned that by improving nervous system function in the process, my team and I can help people with hundreds of different ailments other than back pain. That's what makes me excited to get out of bed every morning.

In the chapters ahead, I'll reveal how what you are doing now for back pain is probably not only wasting your time, but also compounding the problem by making your issues harder to fix and potentially costing you years of your life. You will learn where back pain really comes from, what you can do to end it, and how you can keep it from coming back once and for all. You will take away from this book a plan of action and a future filled with hope.

Finally, you will likely be angry with the current "system," but you will have the facts to never again be a victim of propaganda designed to enrich the pharmaceutical companies and hospitals at your expense. Want proof? Look no further than America's opioid crisis, which has been inextricably linked to the Purdue Pharma manufacturing of OxyContin, a pain drug that has the same basic composition and induces the same euphoric effects as heroin. The drugmaker lied about OxyContin's addictiveness and chose profits over the lives of millions of Americans. In fact, the company enticed physicians to overprescribe the drugs and create de facto drug dens by unscrupulous pharmacies. These are the same physicians no one would ever suspect of "selling out." And even though the crisis was easy to see, Purdue continued to make tens of billions of dollars every year.

These kinds of activities aren't isolated to drugs like OxyContin. It's a game that is being played at the highest levels in corporate pharma and the government that is supposed to protect us, with backdoor deals, questionable payoffs, and conflicts of interest. A game in which some of the FDA members are stockholders in the same companies they should be protecting us from. It makes you ask yourself, "Is there a better way?"

The answer is profoundly "yes."

In the pages ahead, you will find the how-to guide of nonsurgical solutions for handling your back and neck pain. If you follow my recommendations, in just a few weeks you'll be saying what thousands of our patients have said for twenty years: "Why didn't anybody ever tell me this before?"

Yours in health,
Dr. Bradford Butler

For more information on living an exceptional life, free of pain, go to drbradfordbutler.com and sign up for our newsletter on living a longer, happier, and healthier life.

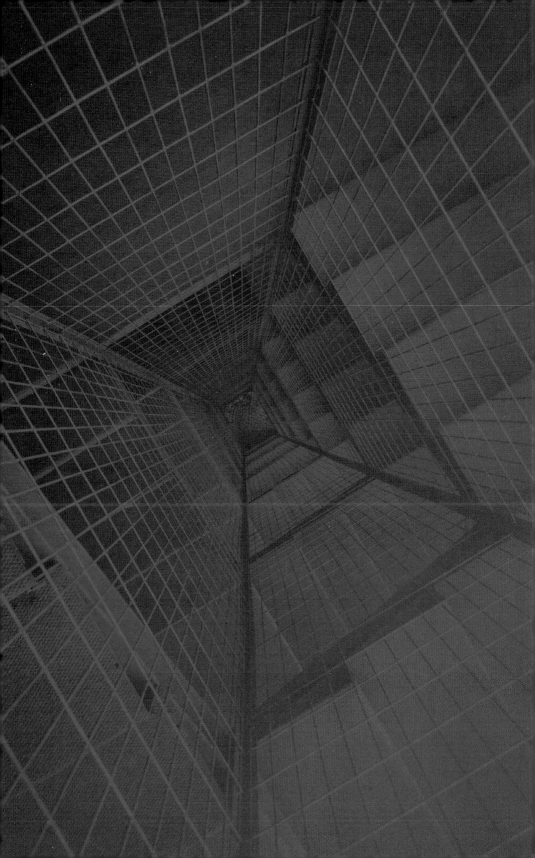

CHAPTER ONE

WHAT YOU DON'T KNOW WILL HURT YOU

Imagine this scenario: You wake up with a painful, swollen mouth. You can't chew your food, you can't drink anything hot or cold without agonizing pain. Clearly there's something wrong; there's got to be a reason for your pain.

So, you call and set up an appointment with your dentist. He examines your mouth and sure enough, you've got a huge cavity—the damage goes all the way down into the nerve. What do you think would happen next? Logically, he would repair the cavity and in a day or so, you would feel as good as new.

But what if he didn't repair the cavity? What if he told you that to help you feel better he was just going to give you a lot of powerful drugs, maybe even an injection, and then send you on your way? That makes no sense, right? It would be ridiculous for the dentist to give you medication to numb the pain and to not fix what's causing it. Left untreated, the pain would get more debilitating and the damage to the tooth would worsen, leading to bigger and more invasive and expensive procedures—a downward spiral.

But that's exactly what happens when it comes to the American health care system and back pain treatment. Our current system only treats the symptoms of back pain; it does not fix the problem. It's no wonder you still have pain; no one has addressed what's causing it.

SHOULD YOU TRUST THE HEALTH CARE SYSTEM?

A lot of decisions doctors make are not based on the patient's best interests; they're based on what procedure can get approved for payment by an insurance provider. One example is spinal fusion surgery. It's commonly believed that spinal fusion surgery "may work" 25 to 50 percent of the time. In reality, the surgery fails the vast majority of the time.[1] But you wouldn't know that by the ads that display when you Google "back pain." Yet surgery rates have increased sixfold since the late 2000s. Why? Maybe it's because a surgeon can charge over $100,000 for the procedure.[2]

Medical doctors are very reluctant to recommend nonmedical treatments, because those are outside of their schooling and the allopathic method of mainstream medicine. Translation: MDs don't even know what they don't know.

Here's the typical cycle: A person has back pain. They try to wait, or they use over-the-counter medications, hoping the pain will go away, but neither helps. So they go to their primary care doctor.

---

1   J.C. Smith, "Back Surgery: Too Many, Too Costly and Too Ineffective," *To Your Health* 5, no. 6 (June 2011), accessed July 25, 2017, http://toyourhealth.com/mpacms/tyh/article.php?id=1447.

2   "Spinal Fusion Surgery Worth the Cost for Stenosis Patients?" Spine-health.com, accessed August 2, 2017, https://www.spine-health.com/blog/spinal-fusion-surgery-worth-cost-stenosis-patients.

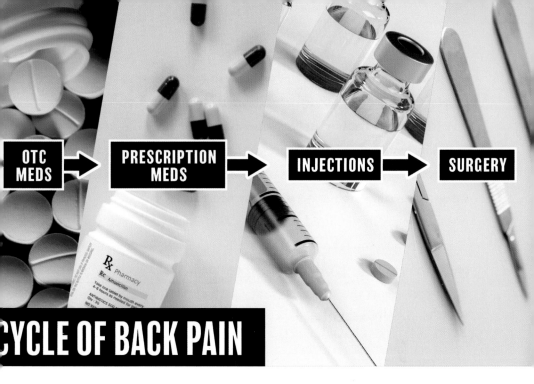

OTC
MEDS

PRESCRIPTION
MEDS

INJECTIONS

SURGERY

CYCLE OF BACK PAIN

The primary care doctor then prescribes stronger prescription drugs, but these don't help either. Over time, the primary care doctor refers the patient out to a pain management doctor or a neurologist who does spinal injections or epidurals. These don't help either—the only course of action remaining is to recommend surgery.

Where are you currently in this cycle?

TAKE CHARGE OF YOUR HEALTH

At some point, you must look at a failed system and ask: "Why?" When it comes to back pain, blind faith in any doctor is not the answer. Instead, ask yourself, "If I go to a doctor who claims to be able to help me, what is he or she trained to do?"

In the primary care world, doctors are simply trained to analyze and then treat the symptoms. For example, if you have pain, they want to address the pain. Therefore, it should come as no surprise when they do what they are supposed to do for pain, which is give you a drug. The purpose of the drug is not to correct the problem causing the pain, but only to mask the symptoms—to reduce the pain.

The same holds true when you see a surgeon. Ask yourself, "What is in this surgeon's bag of tricks?" Well, surgery, of course. Again, it should come as no surprise when you go to a surgeon and he or she suggests you need surgery, because that's what they do.

So how do you take charge of your health when it comes to back pain? Look at what gives the best bang for the buck with the least downside—that's the advice I give my patients.

Consider these statistics: [3]

- Spinal surgery can cost up to $150,000, yet its success rates are only 25 to 50 percent. On top of that, surgery comes with a lot of pain and months of rehabilitation before you realize that it didn't work.

- Recent research shows that medications not only don't work, but they often lead to other health problems such as addiction or ruining your liver.

Why do we, as Americans, have this chronic-treatment view of health care? Because we are taught to. In the United States, we spend more than double on health care what the next country on the list spends. Yet when it comes to quality of care, we are near the bottom in virtually every survey of industrialized nations. In 2016, we were fiftieth out of fifty-five countries in life expectancy, behind some countries many

---

3   J.C. Smith, "Back Surgery: Too Many, Too Costly and Too Ineffective," *To Your Health* 5, no. 6 (June 2011), accessed July 25, 2017, http://toyourhealth.com/mpacms/tyh/article.php?id=1447.

would consider Third World.[4] The World Health Organization (WHO) ranked the United States thirty-seventh at keeping our citizens healthy.[5] And a Time.com report ranked the US health care system as worst among all industrialized nations when it comes to "efficiency, equity and outcomes."[6] Why would you want to follow a system that is, quite frankly, the worst at delivering the results you need and want?

If you were to decide today who controls your health care choices, would you choose a system that is clearly failing, or would you decide that it's finally time to make your own decisions?

When it comes to treatment, the current US health care model tells you what to do without providing all the facts. However, this model ends up employing the costliest, most invasive, and least successful treatments first. When those treatments ultimately fail and your trust in the doctor is broken, you're left to hope that by some miracle there is still a treatment that will work—until then, you're stuck in an endless loop of chronic treatment.

As a doctor and a practical person, what bothers me the most is all the time patients spend having unnecessary and ineffective care. All that wasted time allows for conditions to get worse and makes it harder for my team and I to employ treatments that really do work. All that wasted time pursuing ineffective treatments could have instead been used to heal.

---

4   Lisa Du and Wei Lu, "U.S. Health-Care System Ranks as One of the Least-Efficient," Bloomberg, September 28, 2016, accessed August 3, 2017, https://www.bloomberg.com/news/articles/2016-09-29/u-s-health-care-system-ranks-as-one-of-the-least-efficient.

5   "World Health Organization's Ranking of the World's Health Systems," The Patient Factor, accessed August 3, 2017, http://thepatientfactor.com/canadian-health-care-information/world-health-organizations-ranking-of-the-worlds-health-systems.

6   Melissa Hellman, "U.S. Health Care Ranked Worst in the Developed World," Time.com, June 16, 2014, accessed August 3, 2017, http://time.com/2888403/u-s-health-care-ranked-worst-in-the-developed-world. ·

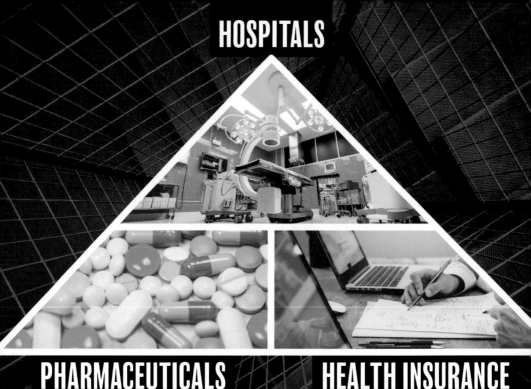

HOSPITALS

PHARMACEUTICALS

HEALTH INSURANCE

MEDICINE IS BIG BUSINESS

Recently on *Fox News*, commentator Steve Hilton of *The Next Revolution* described the behemoth cartel that medicine has become. He drew a diagram of what he called a "Health Swamp Triangle," with the three points of the triangle representing pharma, hospitals, and government.[7] That is the big business model patients are caught in. Hospitals are now big corporations and conglomerates that are run like Fortune 500 companies, with boards, CEOs, and a focus on profits. Drug companies are manufacturing and promoting drugs, with money—not your health—in mind. Years ago, they were not even allowed to advertise, but through successful lobbying efforts (payoffs and bribes), they convinced the FDA to allow what is now

---

7   Steve Hilton, "Swamp Watch: Health care and pharmaceuticals," "The Next Revolution" segment on *Fox News*, July 9, 2017 (online clip), 8:36, http://video. foxnews.com/v/5499431447001/?#sp=show-clips.

called direct-to-consumer (DTC) advertising, which was made legal in 1985.[8] Giving drug companies unlimited access to our minds, with billions of dollars going to high-profile advertising agencies to create sometimes misleading or false claims, has led to unprecedented profits in the drug industry.

In fact, a study by the Kaiser Family Foundation found that every "additional dollar spent on DTC advertising in 2000 yielded $4.20 in additional pharmaceutical sales that year."[9] That's more than a four-to-one return on investment. In 2009, WHO reported that Pfizer, in an effort to make significant profits on Lipitor, its anti-cholesterol drug, created a $260 million advertising campaign. The campaign featured "the inventor of the artificial heart" stating, "Just because I'm a doctor doesn't mean I don't worry about my cholesterol." The man then went on to recommend Lipitor. Here's the problem: Pfizer lied. The man in the campaign is not a doctor; he couldn't write a prescription for anyone, and according to former colleagues he did not invent the artificial heart in the first place.[10]

According to the WHO report, critics of DTC advertising doubt its intent to inform patients. Instead, DTC advertising targets people who are suffering from a disease and seeks to drive their choice to a specific product. And because of this mind-control tactic, as one critic states, "It's much more likely that general practitioners will just do what the patient asks."[11] Drug companies know that's how their

---

8   "Direct-to-consumer advertising under fire," *Bulletin of the World Health Organization* 87, no. 8 (August 2009): 565–644, accessed July 25, 2017, http://www.who.int/bulletin/volumes/87/8/09-040809/en/.

9   "Impact of Direct-to-Consumer Advertising on Prescription Drug Spending," The Henry J. Kaiser Family Foundation (June 2003), 2.

10 "Direct-to-consumer advertising under fire," *Bulletin of the World Health Organization* 87, no. 8 (August 2009): 565–644, accessed July 25, 2017, http://www.who.int/bulletin/volumes/87/8/09-040809/en/.

11 Ibid.

advertising works, so they continue to pour more and more dollars into influencing you and your thinking.

Then there's the United States Food & Drug Administration (FDA), an agency of the United States Department of Health and Human Services. The role of the FDA is to protect you as a citizen and the public at large by assuring the safety, efficacy, and security of products that are sold to you. That includes pharmaceuticals.

But there's a major flaw here. It's called "lobbying." For many years now, there have been reports that the drug companies are in the pockets of some of the very people charged with protecting US consumers. The result is that drugs that are not safe or effective—and that are sometimes even deadly—sneak through the system and are released for public consumption. That should *never* happen.

One example of a drug that should never have made it into the hands of consumers is Vioxx, a powerful nonsteroidal anti-inflammatory drug (NSAID). After being approved by the FDA and then released into the market in 2000, hundreds of thousands of prescriptions were written for the drug. This happened even though some in the medical community warned about the potentially deadly effects of Vioxx before its release. In the end, it took four years—during which sixty thousand people died from heart-related side effects— before Vioxx was pulled from the market.[12]

How can something like that happen in America? Well, just follow the money trail. There are significant conflicts of interest between FDA members and their business relationships with Big Pharma. Here are some facts uncovered in a 2014 study of the voting behaviors and reported financial interests of nearly fourteen hundred

12 "NSAIDs: The Painful Truth Behind Painkillers Infographic," Mercola.com, accessed August 2, 2017, http://www.mercola.com/infographics/nsaids.htm.

advisory committee members of the FDA Center for Drug Evaluation Research.[13]

- Thirteen percent of members in any given FDA committee had financial interests in the company whose drugs were up for review.

- About one-third consulted for a drugmaker.

- One-fourth had ownership interests.

- Sixty-three percent of the time, members with financial ties to that company voted in favor of the drug.

- Committee members who served on sponsoring firms' advisory boards had an 84 percent chance of voting in favor of the drug's approval.[14]

Unfortunately, the same kinds of conflict of interest occur between the prescribing doctors and the drug firms.[15] Drug companies are notorious for using principles of influence with MDs, and statistics overwhelmingly show that when a drug company provides a doctor with a gift of some kind (trips, lunches, research grants, company shares, and other goodies), the doctor's prescribing behaviors are typically affected. Among the studies was one that reported on physicians who had been

---

13 Genevieve Pham-Kanter, "Revisiting Financial Conflicts of Interest in FDA Advisory Committees," The Milbank Quarterly, September 2014, accessed August 2, 2017, https://www.milbank.org/quarterly/articles/revisiting-financial-conflicts-of-interest-in-fda-advisory-committees/.

14 Aaron Carroll, "Doctors' Magical Thinking About Conflicts of Interest," *The New York Times*, September 8, 2014, accessed August 2, 2017, https://www.nytimes.com/2014/09/09/upshot/doctors-magical-thinking-about-conflicts-of-interest.html?partner=rss&emc=rss&_r=2&abt=0002&abg=0.

15 Ibid.

to new-drug symposia with all expenses paid; although 85 percent of physicians interviewed said gifts wouldn't influence them, after the meeting, the prescription rates for the featured drugs tripled.[16]

One of the more frightening physician ties to Big Pharma surfaced in 2015, when Robert Califf, MD, a vice chancellor at Duke University, was nominated to be commissioner of the FDA, a position he ultimately held throughout 2016. As reported in a 2015 *Time* article, Califf had "close ties to big pharma."[17] In fact, Califf reportedly openly admitted to NPR: "Many of us consult with the pharmaceutical industry, which I think is a very good thing. They need ideas, and then the decision about what they do is really up to the person who is funding the study." Seriously? Yes, he said that. In fact, Dr. Califf is known for defending Vioxx, the same drug that resulted in sixty thousand deaths.[18]

During his career at Duke, Califf received money from twenty-three different drug companies (Johnson & Johnson, Merck, Lilly, GSK, and others), some of which he served in roles such as director, officer, partner, advisor, consultant.[19] In other words, he was and is in their pockets. How can the FDA be trusted when someone like Califf could head the organization?

Further, the FDA model for drug testing is completely flawed. The *Time* article stated that "The FDA uses a model for drug testing and oversight largely developed in the early 1960s." The model

---

16 "Conflicts of Interest Rampant Among FDA Advisors, Study Shows," Mercola. com, September 24, 2014, accessed August 2, 2017, http://articles.mercola.com/ sites/articles/archive/2014/09/24/fda-advisors-drug-approval-decisions.aspx.

17 Massimo Calabresi, "Candidate to Lead FDA Has Close Ties to Big Pharma," *Time*, accessed August 2, 2017, http://www.time.com/3714242/ candidate-to-lead-fda-has-close-ties-to-big-pharma.

18 Martha Rosenberg, "The FDA Now Officially Belongs to Big Pharma," Alternet. org, February 24, 2016, accessed August 2, 2017, http://www.alternet.org/ news-amp-politics/fda-now-officially-belongs-big-pharma.

19 Ibid.

essentially allows the drug companies to do their own research to prove their drug is safe and effective. Then, after providing their own research to the FDA (no conflict there, right?), the drugmakers can market and sell the drug to the public and then continue to monitor the safety after it's already being sold, essentially using the American people as guinea pigs. If the drug doesn't kill too many people, then the drugmaker can continue to sell it.

In fact, due to this inherent flaw, adverse reactions to drugs are still a leading cause of death in the United States.[20] Medical error, a category that includes adverse drug reactions, is the third leading cause.[21]

ARE DRUGS AND SURGERY YOUR ANSWER TO BACK PAIN RELIEF?

The research is in and indicates that *no*, drugs and surgery are not the answer to back pain relief. Not only are they not shown to be effective, but the costs related to them are staggering. Research is showing that there are more than 650,000 spinal surgeries per year at a cost of over $20 billion.[22] That is a huge financial incentive for surgeons to perform surgery. Sadly, research also shows that as many as 90 percent are ineffective or unnecessary.[23]

---

20   "The FDA Exposed," Mercola.com, accessed August 2, 2017, http://www. mercola.com/Downloads/bonus/the-FDA-exposed/default.aspx.

21   "Medical Errors: STILL the Third Leading Cause of Death," Mercola. com, accessed July 26, 2017, http://articles.mercola.com/sites/articles/ archive/2016/05/18/medical-errors-death.aspx.

22   "Spinal Fusion Surgery Worth the Cost for Stenosis Patients?" accessed August 2, 2017, https://www.spine-health.com/blog/ spinal-fusion-surgery-worth-cost-stenosis-patients.

23   J.C. Smith, "Back Surgery: Too Many, Too Costly and Too Ineffective," *To Your Health* 5, no. 6 (June 2011), accessed July 25, 2017, http://toyourhealth.com/ mpacms/tyh/article.php?id=1447.

When you consider that there is an 80 percent chance you will suffer from back pain at some point in your life, it's up to you to decide what does work, and choose to avoid what doesn't.[24]

So where do you go from here? In the coming chapters, I will discuss in-depth where back pain comes from and how you, as the key decision maker for your health, need to think about your back pain if you want to get better and not be another victim of bad choice.

---

24   Ibid.

TAKE IT ←··OR··→ LEAVE IT

- This book is designed to lay out the facts and opinions you need to know to make the best choice for your health.

- As Americans, we are blessed with some of the best doctors in the world. However, our system is so corrupt and profit driven that you, the patient, must question everything your doctors recommend. Your treatment must make sense to you.

- Our health care system is backward, and it's rigged against you, the patient. It has conditioned people to look for the quick fix by the medical-pharmaceutical complex. As a result, people are convinced to choose the most dangerous and invasive procedures and treatments first, even though they deliver the worst results.

- You need to wake up. If you don't think health care fails can happen to you, you're wrong.

- It's my personal mission to change how Americans think about their spines and how they deal with their back pain. Reading this book is the first step.

Visit drbradfordbutler.com for more information.

- 𝕏 **@dr_bbutler**
- f **www.facebook.com/drbradfordbutler**
- in **www.linkedin.com/in/dr-brad-butler**

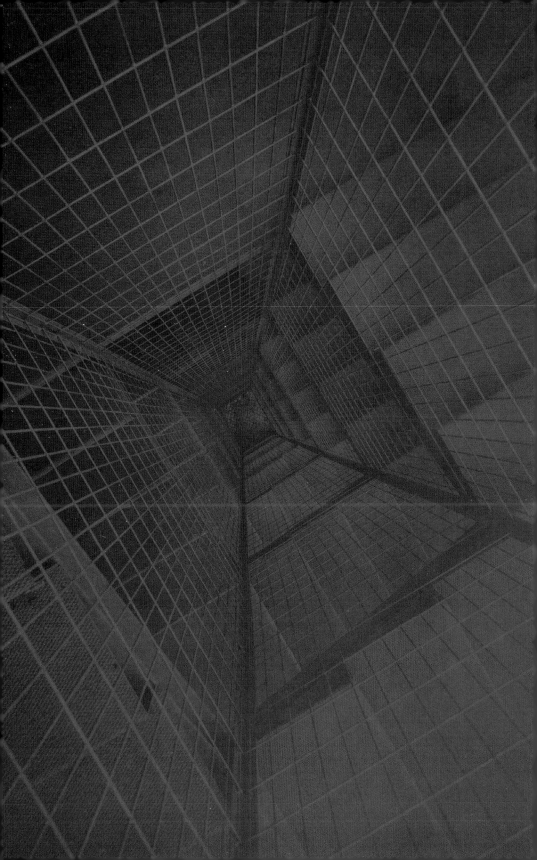

CHAPTER TWO
THE "REAL" COSTS OF BACK PAIN

In the last chapter, I discussed the physical and financial costs of the corrupt and ineffective system we in America call "health care." But those costs pale in comparison to the emotional and psychological costs of back pain for a patient stripped of all hope. In all of my years helping people, I've seen that the emotional costs are always the most debilitating.

It's such an important part of the equation that I'm asking you now the same question I've asked my patients for over a decade: "What things do you love in life that you can no longer do because of the pain?"

Every patient we see at my clinics tells us the same thing: they want to get rid of their pain. But the real reason they come is because of what the pain is stopping them from doing. That's what really matters to them. Whether it's gardening, dancing, sports, walking, sitting and watching TV, playing with or holding their children and grandchildren, you name it, they want that back.

People don't come to see me and my team just because they want to be numb to their pain. There are lots of ways to do that, I might

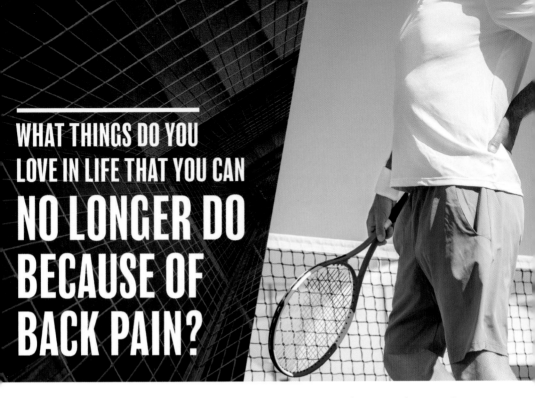

WHAT THINGS DO YOU LOVE IN LIFE THAT YOU CAN NO LONGER DO BECAUSE OF BACK PAIN?

add—both legally and illegally. They come to us because the pain has stopped them from functioning in life, and there's a real emotional cost to not being able to function. That cost manifests in fear, insecurity, anxiety, and even depression.

Yes, depression is one of the outcomes of pain. In many patients, it's chronic pain that leads to a diagnosis of depression. According to the Mayo Clinic, "Chronic pain causes a number of problems that can lead to depression, such as trouble sleeping and stress."[25] Over the years, many patients have told us that when they finally started feeling better, they also experienced dramatic reductions in their feelings of stress, anxiety, and depression.

One patient of mine, Joe, experienced just such a dramatic turnaround, but I really understood the impact when his wife, Sandra,

---

25   Daniel K. Hall-Flavin, "Pain and depression: Is there a link?" Mayo Clinic, accessed July 26, 2017,
http://www.mayoclinic.org/diseases-conditions/depression/expert-answers/
pain-and-depression/faq-20057823.

reached out to me with a wonderful thank-you note. After many years of failed medical treatment, Joe completely recovered from his symptoms—he no longer had chronic pain. In her note, Sandra thanked me and my team for giving her back her husband, and her marriage.

Have you considered how your pain is robbing you of your life? Sadly, too many patients are misdiagnosed with depression and put on very powerful and dangerous medications because of pain. It's as if their doctor grew tired of not having answers and finally concluded that "it must all be in their head." Unable to resolve their patient's pain, the doctor just ends up writing a prescription for depression medication.

A 2004 article from the *Primary Care Companion to the Journal of Clinical Psychiatry* seems to confirm the situation. The article states, "A high percentage of patients with depression who seek treatment in a primary care setting report *only physical symptoms…*" (emphasis added).[26] In other words, the doctors can't prove it, but they want to classify you as depressed because you're in pain. They're trying to say that it's the depression that gives you physical pain, when it's the pain that causes the depression. Again, the problem is that they have no solution for the pain, but they do have lots of drugs. "So let's diagnose you with a condition that we can prescribe something for" seems to be the general consensus. As I mentioned in chapter one, it's all backwards and corrupt.

The real cost of back pain—the emotional toll it takes—isn't reserved solely for the average patient either. Plenty of celebrities have

---

26 Madhukar Trivedi, "The Link Between Depression and Physical Symptoms," *The Primary Care Companion to the Journal of Clinical Psychiatry*, suppl.1, no. 6 (2004):12-16, accessed July 26, 2017, on U.S. National Library of Medicine, National Institutes of Health, https://www.ncbi.nlm.nih.gov/pmc/articles/PMC486942/.

fallen victim to the allure of the quick fix (drugs and surgery)—and it costs them dearly. There are too many to mention, but in recent times, the news has reported on problems resulting from drugs and failed surgeries involving Tiger Woods, Matthew Perry, Jamie Lee Curtis, Michael Jackson, and Charlie Sheen, to name a few.

As I was putting together my thoughts for this book, two extremely well known basketball coaches—Steve Kerr of the Golden State Warriors and Thad Matta of the Ohio State Buckeyes—were in the news because of their failed surgeries. Kerr was even quoted as saying, "Stay away from back surgery."[27] And Matta is still angry after a botched surgery in 2007 left him wearing a brace for life and with a permanent disability in his right foot.[28]

Think about it: These celebrities have almost unlimited resources, and their names give them access to "the best doctors in the business." So if having money, celebrity status, and the best doctors and hospitals can't help someone with back pain get better, then maybe the methods they're using just don't work.

Look at the cost to the lives of these people—and that's just a fraction of the total. Many people have had their lives ripped apart by back surgery and drugs, leading to divorce, lost jobs, bankruptcy, and for some, even death.

You see, the real cost of back pain is so much more than most people realize. It ruins lives every day.

---

27 Tracy Seipel, "Is Warriors Coach Kerr's 'stay away from surgery' advice the right call?," *The Mercury News*, April 24, 2017, accessed July 26, 2017, http://www.mercurynews.com/2017/04/24/ is-warriors-coach-kerrs-stay-away-from-surgery-good-advice/.

28 Mike Leprestl, "The things he can't do: Matta's health concerns, and why he's still coaching," NCAA.com, March 16, 2015, accessed July 26, 2017, http://www. ncaa.com/news/basketball-men/article/2015-03-16/things-he-cant-do.

TIME IS YOUR BEST FRIEND OR YOUR BIGGEST ENEMY

One of the critical yet missed components of this entire equation is the role that time plays.

Most of the people I've mentioned, and the science I've been citing, revolves around chronic back pain.

It's chronic back pain—and I emphasize *chronic*—that affects 80 percent of Americans in their lives. "Chronic" is defined by Merriam-Webster as "continuing or occurring again and again for a long time."

But there's another definition by Merriam-Webster that can more accurately describe what it means to have "chronic" back pain: "growing stronger and firmer with time so as to resist change or reform."

In other words, the way I want you to view the back/time connection is that the longer you have a back problem—whether it's mild or severe—the more damage it will create, the more it will "resist getting better," and the more time it will take to heal.

In fact, keep in mind that when it comes to back pain, *there is a point of no return*. There may come a time when there's nothing that anyone can do to overcome the damage you have *allowed* to occur by waiting too long.

That's what happened to Barry, a patient who came to see me several years ago after he had already taken the traditional, albeit incorrect route for his back pain. The reason he tried the traditional route was that he only had mild lower back pain, right below the belt line (known as the lumbosacral junction). He had lived with the pain for several years, but it had come and gone, and the episodes were never really severe. Over the years, when he had an episode of back pain, he would just take some over-the-counter medication for a few days until it went away. However, in the year prior to his consult with me, the pain had become more frequent and the duration of each episode was longer. And he was starting to get some numbness and tingling in his left foot.

He had heard about us, like most of our patients, because of our reputation for getting results. Prior to seeing us, he went to his traditional doctor, who labeled his foot numbness and tingling as neuropathy. Neuropathy has been linked with certain diseases, such as diabetes, but it's just a description rather than a diagnosis. To patients it's just a big word, but technically what it describes is "a problem with the nerves." (Earth shattering, right?)

Among the most common causes of neuropathy is long-term compression or pressure on the nerve roots as they exit the spine and head toward the foot. When we examined Barry, that's exactly what we found. He was about sixty-five years of age, and he'd had a very sedentary job his whole life. The result of all those years of sitting was significant deterioration of his lower spine and discs along with structural alignment issues where his vertebrae were twisting and curving when they should be aligned.

After examining Barry, I told him that the news was good and bad. The good news was that we could help him and that we had an incredible success rate for cases like his. The bad news was that his problem had been building for a long time (there's that word "time" again) and was therefore chronic. That meant it would take around twelve weeks of advanced care using a system I created known as the "Butler Spine Program." I'll discuss the details of this revolutionary approach to spinal care in chapter 7.

The key to the program's success is in combining multiple therapies and disciplines in each treatment, which allows the entire area around the condition to heal.

Unfortunately, Barry refused my recommendation. He told me that he didn't want to commit to the time and money necessary to invest in his recovery. So, he left my office and went back to his traditional doctor, who put him on drugs to treat the symptoms.

The story, unfortunately, doesn't end there. Almost exactly two years later, Barry returned to my office, only this time he was only able to walk with the aid of a walker. In the two years since I had seen him, his condition had continued to worsen. His back pain was severe at that point, and it had spread to his hips. His left foot was completely numb, and the neuropathy had migrated to his right foot. His health was a mess.

As it turned out, over time, the drugs the doctor had prescribed were no longer effective, so he had begun a series of injections—none of them worked. So over time his failure to properly address the problem allowed the degenerating spine to continue breaking down.

By the time he came to see me, he was in the midst of consulting with surgeons who—you guessed it—all told him that surgery was his only hope.

Now, maybe you expect me to tell you that, like Superman, we swooped in and saved the day for Barry—that we put him through the twelve-week program and, magically, he fully recovered! Unfortunately, that's not what happened—we do great work, but we're not superheroes.

After examining Barry again, we found that in the two years he waited, the spine had decayed so much that it was unlikely we could still help him. I had to tell him I could no longer accept his case. To this day, I remember quite vividly the moment I told him, because I could see the light drain from his eyes.

Of course, had Barry followed my recommendations two years earlier, it is very likely he would have had a full recovery and gotten

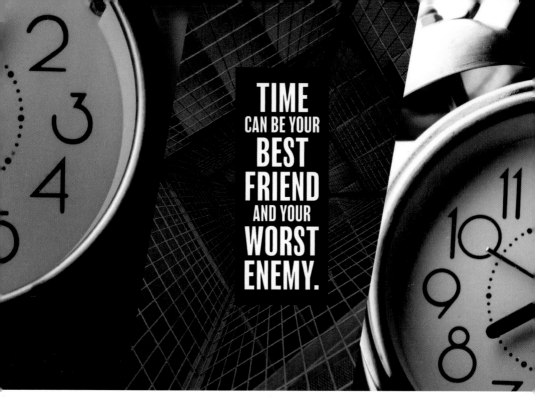

TIME CAN BE YOUR BEST FRIEND AND YOUR WORST ENEMY.

his life back. But he had come back to us as a last resort, and by then it was too late. I never heard from him again, but I can only imagine that he remained disabled for the rest of his life.

Barry's story bothers me every time I share it, because it didn't have to happen that way. But that's what it means to be accountable for your health and to understand the facts behind your conditions along with the consequences of your choices. His story epitomizes what I mean when I say: *time* can be your best friend or your worst enemy.

THE DENTAL PROFESSION HAS IT RIGHT

The dental profession is one area of medicine that has evolved incredibly over the last few decades.

My mom was born in the early 1930s, and I remember asking her many years ago, "Mom, when you were a kid, how often did you go to see a dentist?" She replied that no one went to a dentist unless *there was a real problem.* That "real problem" usually resulted in a tooth being pulled. Then I asked her, "So why, when we were kids, did you take us for a checkup every year?" Her response was perfect: "I guess we learned better," she said.

It's true that the dental profession has turned into the "prevention profession" by embarking on a strong campaign about healthy teeth and habits. The results are in, and getting the message out works. Due to proper dental hygiene practices, including checkups to prevent small problems from becoming big ones, we have a country with smiles that are the envy of the world. In the United States, people are now smart enough to know that, even without dental pain, it's important to get to the dentist on a regular basis. And when there's even a little bit of pain, it's time to get to the dentist right away. That's the way to prevent small problems from becoming big ones.

That's the way it needs to be for neck and back pain. At our offices, we are making that same practice of regular checkups and visits at the first sign of pain a reality for neck and back pain sufferers.

When a patient comes to my office, it isn't enough to just relieve their pain. Being free of symptoms, just like in dentistry, doesn't mean you don't have major problems brewing. It just means that you don't know that they're developing. That's why we educate our patients on the fact that symptoms only come after there's a problem that's been uncorrected for so long, and symptoms are usually the first thing to go away, long before the real problem is fixed.

In other words, symptoms are the last piece of the problem to develop, and the first to disappear.

Yes, we still must address the pain, which we do with state-of-the-art technology that—unlike popping pills or undergoing surgery—has no side effects. Instead, the technology works with the body's natural mechanism to reduce pain and inflammation. That buys time to combine other traditional therapies to stimulate the body to heal and repair itself. That's the way treating back pain is supposed to be done.

In the next few chapters, you will learn more about where your pain is really coming from and how to craft a plan to win the game.

TAKE IT ←··OR··→ LEAVE IT

- It's likely that your back pain isn't going to just cost you time. By ignoring it and not fixing the underlying problem, you are destined to suffer a much worse fate than you should.

- The psychological costs of pain are immense. Left untreated, chronic pain can lead to emotional issues, including depression. In fact, most depression patients may be misdiagnosed. It might be the psychological effect of chronic pain that was left untreated.

- Back surgery and prescription drugs are almost always the wrong choice. Many patients who use these options don't need them, and the ones who do have staggeringly high failure rates.

- Education is the key. You are responsible for your choices, not your doctor. Question how the treatment plans he or she recommends will help you and how it will correct what's causing the pain, not merely mask it.

- Don't waste time. *It will never be easier, faster, or cheaper to fix your back pain than today.* The longer you wait, the more damage and degeneration will occur, making it harder and taking longer to get relief, often at a higher cost to you.

Visit drbradfordbutler.com for more information.

- ⓨ **@dr_bbutler**
- ⓕ **www.facebook.com/drbradfordbutler**
- ⓘⓝ **www.linkedin.com/in/dr-brad-butler**

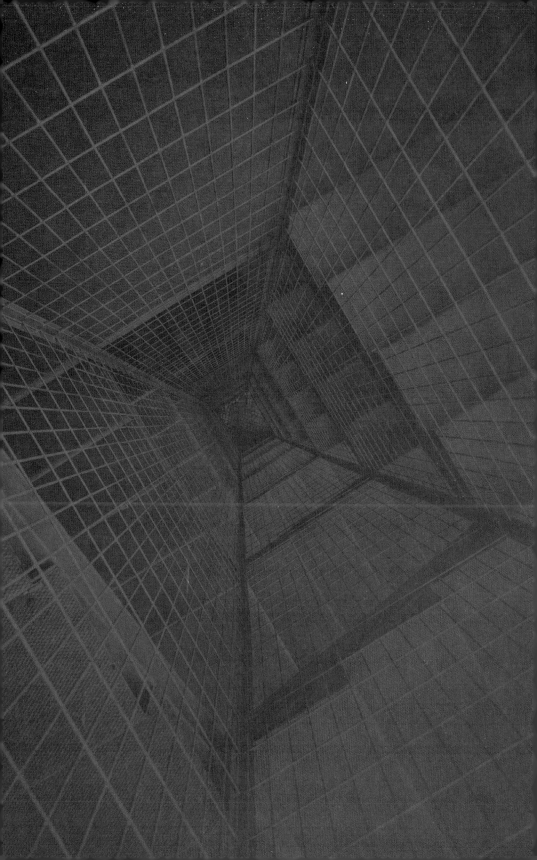

CHAPTER THREE

IS IT TOO LATE FOR *YOUR* BACK OR IS HEALING AN INSIDE JOB?

S o, is it time to give up? No, never—never give up. The future is bright as long as my team and I work to educate people about how the older, more traditional therapies work and about emerging science and research on alternatives to drugs and surgery.

You may have been told by your doctor that you must live with your pain, but that couldn't be further from the truth. Our motto at Oakland Spine & Physical Therapy is "No Drugs, No Surgery—Just Results."

  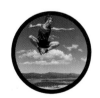

No Drugs.   No Surgery.   **Just Results.**

Hope for a better future may mean a change in mindset, a change in your own belief system. In America, when it comes to health, people often live by the credo: "If it ain't broke, don't fix it." Or perhaps even worse, they believe in the quick fix, the "Band Aid approach" to treating health problems. The American culture is one that believes that sickness comes from outside the body. The germ theory of disease, for instance, holds that bad bacteria and micro-organisms invade the body and that's what causes you to get sick. Similarly, our culture believes that getting healthy also must come from outside the body—by taking pills or undergoing surgery. But if you take a moment to think about the situation logically, you will see that none of that really makes sense. If everyone got sick simply because of germs, we'd all be sick all the time. There are no more germs (bacteria) on a person when they are sick than when they are healthy, are there?

The truth is that *sick* people get sick. In other words, you only get sick when your body can't adapt to the changing environment, when your immune system can't fight off germs when it needs to. Remember my story in the Introduction to this book about how I got into chiropractic? I talked about how health is defined by the presence of function in your organs and systems. It's not defined by feeling good or bad.

When your immune system is functioning normally, you don't get sick. When I was a child, no one asked *why* I kept getting sick until my chiropractor suggested that because of my spine, I probably had a weak immune system. After a few weeks of care, I didn't get sick anymore, regardless of the germs.

The same holds true with back pain. In a healthy, functioning person, the body repairs damage as it occurs. There are specific cells in the body designed to destroy old, worn-out tissues while other cells grow new, healthy tissues.

When your body is healthy, that tissue repair goes on day and night under the control of your brain and nervous system. However, if your body isn't functioning properly, it can't replace the degenerating tissues fast enough. Old tissue begins to slowly accumulate, and over many years you develop enough damaged tissue to cause a real problem. With back pain, that buildup usually is happening to multiple tissues at the same time. Again, the symptoms only occur after the damage has happened. You don't get symptoms beforehand.

Another problem is that as people age, their pain threshold grows, which allows for more and more damage to develop before symptoms arise.

I explain to my patients that your "pain threshold" is like a thermostat for damage. Your pain threshold operates a lot like a thermostat in your home. For example, if it's fifty degrees outside and you have your thermostat set at eighty degrees, your heat will kick on until it reaches that eighty degree threshold. Once the temperature exceeds eighty degrees, your thermostat will trigger your cooling system to kick on. The house will then cool until it reaches that eighty degree thermostat setting.

The nervous system works in a similar manner. It won't trigger prematurely. Otherwise we'd all be in pain all the time. Instead, there's a "threshold" or "allowance" for how much damage your nervous system will tolerate before signaling pain. As a person gets older, it's as if someone is raising the temperature setting on a thermostat, meaning it takes even more "heat" to trigger the cooling system. Similarly, with the nervous system, it allows more and more damage to occur before triggering a warning that something is wrong. In this case, that warning is back pain.

So, when it comes to your back and neck, you must change what you believe about caring for your pain. You should view your health from the same perspective as you do your teeth. That means getting in to see the doctor as soon as you sense discomfort. Some people mistakenly think that if they wait and the pain goes away, that means the problem went away. In most cases, only the pain went, not the problem that caused it.

Healing from back pain is like healing from anything else. It's an "inside job." Healing and repair can never come from the outside. That is where the medical system has tricked us all, spending billions to convince people that a pill or a procedure is the path to health. The truth is, medicine can't heal. It can only treat the symptoms.

Think about it this way: When you break a bone, is it the cast that heals you? The pain medication you're prescribed? Or does healing come from your own body? When you cut your finger or bite your tongue, is it something outside of your body that heals the wound? Or is it something from within your body? In all cases, of course, it's your body. So why would back pain be any different? It's not. All you have to do is help the body heal itself.

FIX FIRST, THEN MAINTAIN

The key to your recovery and long-term happiness comes down to what I call "fix first, then maintain." There are two critical concepts here. The first is that you cannot maintain what's broken; it must be fixed first. The second is that after you fix it, if you don't maintain it, you will potentially end up back where you started.

Think about fitness as an example. Most people want to be fit, healthy, and feel good, but they know they aren't. Every New Year's Eve, millions of Americans make a "resolution" that they are going to finally do it—they are finally going to get in shape and stay in shape.

The problem is, they want something they aren't willing to work for, so in no time at all, they give up. They quit.

It's widely known in the gym industry that a gym's survival relies on the first two months of every year, when millions of New Year's resolution makers join up but don't keep showing up. The money that gyms make in those first two months must "carry the weight"—pun intended—for the rest of the year. On top of that, gyms can accept many more memberships than they can service, because they know that most of the people that join aren't committed, they're just "interested." And there's a huge difference in the habits of the committed versus the interested.

To get in shape, you first must face the problem—you're fat. (Remember, I'm comparing this to your chronic back pain, so stay with me here.) Fixing fat means you must go to the gym several times a week for many months before you will see sig-

AFTER YOU FIX IT, IF YOU DON'T MAINTAIN IT, YOU WILL POTENTIALLY END UP BACK WHERE YOU STARTED.

nificant change. Once you see a change, you'll still have to go at least three times a week so that your body will continue to "adapt" to what you are doing for it. (Adapt—that's a keyword, so write it down.) Eventually, you'll get to a point where you look and feel great.

Now, the time it takes to go through the process of getting into shape is different for everyone. Some people have more fat and less muscle because they have been out of shape for so many years. Others have just a little bit of extra fat they need to shed. No matter the amount of fat, or damage, eventually everyone can get there, right?

Once you've achieved the fix, then comes the crucial point in long-term happiness: maintenance. It typically takes a minimum amount of effort to maintain your new body. Maybe working out one to two times a week should sustain you. Again, if you don't commit to the maintenance side of the equation, if you completely stop working to stay fit and go back to your old lifestyle, everything will come back—including the fat.

The same thing happens with your back and spine. Over many years of doing things you didn't know were causing problems, your spine began to adapt to them. That led to joint malfunction, poor posture, muscle imbalances, and other dysfunctions that began the process of degeneration that brought you to where you are today.

The point I'm making is this: to fix your back pain, you must commit to what it takes. Your body is controlled by what is called "the law of adaptation." That means it's designed to adapt to whatever you do most frequently, even if what you do is bad for you. Adaptation is one of the major governing laws of your body. That means if you don't exercise, your muscle system adapts to a lack of use, and the muscles atrophy and get weak. When you exercise, your nervous system registers the increased stress on the muscles and directs them to get stronger and bigger.

Your spine is governed by the same principles. When you sit, move the same way repeatedly, slouch, and so forth, your spine adapts to the stresses even though they create structural and functional problems as time goes on. To fix your back problem, we must apply the same principles to reverse the process. That means we must treat you often enough to stimulate your body to adapt back to how a healthy spine looks and functions.

Then, after your spine is functioning great and you feel fantastic, we must come up with a plan to maintain it. Without maintenance care, the same stuff you were doing that caused the condition in the first place will cause the corrected spine to go back to its dysfunctional position. As I tell my patients, "It's unfortunate that we even have to do corrective care, but we have to fix the problem, and then we have to maintain the correction."

Just like the dental industry successfully taught people how to have healthier teeth, if we are successful in helping people learn how to keep their back healthy, maybe we can stop having to fix them and just get into a maintenance mode. But that's going to take an overhaul of the belief system of our culture. That means a better plan and an understanding that our bodies were created with massively intelligent design, and to be healthy, they need to be set free to function the way they were designed.

There is hope for you!

TAKE IT ←··OR··→ LEAVE IT

- Go to www.oaklandspinenj.com/patient-testimonials for testimonials of patients who had lost all hope and were about to give up until they found out about the Butler Spine Program.

- Do the right things, and you will get the right results. That requires you to think differently about your back.

- Health and healing can never come from outside. Healing comes from the inside out; no pill or surgery can ever heal you. Stop trying to swallow your way back to health and to being pain-free. Instead, unleash healing from within.

- No matter what you want or don't want to believe, your body is designed to adapt to what you do to it most often. Anybody can get better if they do the right things often enough and long enough.

Visit drbradfordbutler.com for more information.

- @dr_bbutler
- www.facebook.com/drbradfordbutler
- www.linkedin.com/in/dr-brad-butler

CHAPTER FOUR

WHAT EVERYONE NEEDS TO KNOW ABOUT THEIR "BACK"

Jason came into my office just as we were closing for the day and asked, "Is there a doctor that I can talk to here?" I happened to be standing at the front desk, so I introduced myself.

"Great," Jason said, then proceeded to tell me his concerns. "I just left my orthopedist's office and he told me I need a double hip replacement."

Now, Jason was a roughly fifty-year-old man who by all appearances was in great shape. So, I asked, "Why do you need a double hip replacement?"

"I don't know. I have pain right here," he said, pointing to his hip. "He did all these different tests and studies and then basically told me that's what I need. How is that possible?"

I told him, "I don't have any of the studies, but I'll tell you what I'll do. I'll give you an exam and take some X-rays, and that will give me the information I need to tell you if he's right." If Jason had such severe arthritis that his hip joints were bone-on-bone, then that would show in his X-rays. But I saw nothing of the sort.

Instead, I told him, "Your problem is not in your hips. It's in your pelvis. It's called the sacroiliac joint. This is what we need to treat. I pretty much can guarantee you that within a few weeks, you're going to see a big difference."

As it turned out, Jason had been a runner for thirty-something years. All that wear and tear from running had affected his lower spine and pelvis. Was he a candidate for surgery? Not in the least.

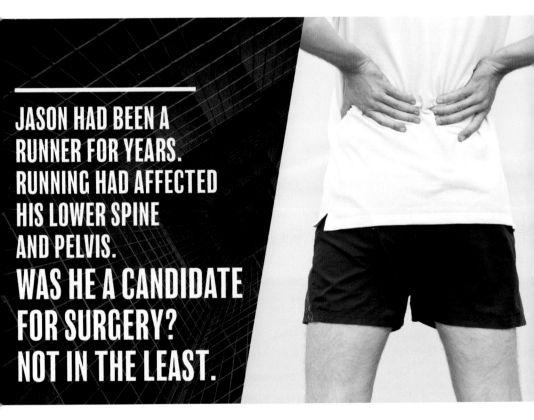

JASON HAD BEEN A RUNNER FOR YEARS. RUNNING HAD AFFECTED HIS LOWER SPINE AND PELVIS. WAS HE A CANDIDATE FOR SURGERY? NOT IN THE LEAST.

We'll come back to Jason's story later on, but the point is that he didn't know where his "hip" pain was really coming from. Do you know where your pain is coming from?

MY "BACK" HURTS

Whenever I meet with a new patient, I always start by asking them about their symptoms, and it is almost guaranteed they will reply that they have "back pain." I then follow their statement with another question, such as "Can you be more specific?" Usually, my question is met with a confused look, and then the patient pointing to an area of their back that's bothering them. "Right around here," they usually say.

While almost every patient reports having "back" pain, where they point varies greatly. One patient may point to the lowest part of their back in the very center. Another may point to their lower back but slightly off-center. Another may point to their hip, and still another may wave their hand over their entire middle back and say, "It's right around this area here."

Why is identifying a specific area of the back so significant? Because everyone knows their "back" as a specific thing. When someone says, "my back hurts," they may be describing anything from their lower back to their mid-back to their upper back, or even their neck. In anatomical terms, the back is just a description of a region.

It's a little like the mouth—everyone can identify their mouth. But when you have pain in your mouth and you want to

THE MORE THAT YOU KNOW ABOUT THE REGION OF YOUR BODY KNOWN AS YOUR BACK, THE MORE SPECIFICALLY YOU CAN HELP YOUR HEALTH CARE PROVIDER UNDERSTAND YOUR PAIN. THEN, THE MORE TARGETED AND SUCCESSFUL YOUR TREATMENT CAN BE.

get it better, it's helpful to understand the structures in the mouth in order to help determine what's causing the pain. Is it a tooth? Is it part of a tooth? Is it the gums? Is the pain coming from the bones that hold the teeth? Is it inflammation in a cheek or in the tongue?

See, the more that you know about the region of your body known as your back, the more specifically you can help your health care provider understand your pain. Then, the more targeted and successful your treatment can be. The best way to fix back or neck pain is to target the source of the pain. If you don't know where your back or neck pain is coming from, then how can you create the best plan for fixing it?

This chapter will help you understand what your back actually is—what makes up the back, what its functions are, and why a healthy back or spine is so critical to your overall health and longevity.

TO BE SPECIFIC, IT'S YOUR SPINE

The most prominent feature of the back, of course, is the spine.

The spine, or backbone, runs from the base of the skull to the pelvis or lower portion of the torso. The spine protects the spinal cord and serves as a pillar of support for the body's weight. In all, your spine consists of twenty-four bones, known as vertebrae, from top to bottom. Each bone allows for movement while protecting the spinal cord as well as the spinal nerves that exist between them. (More on the spinal cord and nerves later.)

The vertebrae are also significant because of the muscles that attach to them. These muscles give the spine a very dynamic ability to move and be flexible. One of the other key functions of your spine is that it allows you to move well when it's healthy and working properly.

Undoubtedly, you have noticed people who don't seem to be in pain but who clearly don't move with ease. What you're seeing is someone who doesn't have a healthy spine even though they don't yet have the symptoms of a bad back. If you or someone you know has abnormal range of motion when walking, moving, turning the head, and so on, that's a warning of future problems.

The spine is made up of three regions: the cervical spine, or neck; the thoracic spine, or mid-back; and the lumbar spine, or lower back. When observed from behind, your spine should be positioned in a straight line from your skull down to your sacrum, or tailbone. That's because your spinal cord hangs straight down from your brain. The spine is in its healthiest position when it is straight.

A side view of the spine, however, reveals that there are three natural opposing curves that give the spine its classic S-shape. These curves help the spine to withstand significant amounts of stress by providing more even bodyweight distribution. From an engineering standpoint, curves can make things stronger. The curves in the neck and lower back have the same shape; these are known as the "lordosis." The curves in the mid-back and the sacrum are called the "kyphosis."

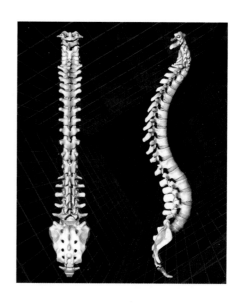

A side view of the spine reveals that there are three natural opposing curves that give the spine its classic S-shape.

In a normally formed and functioning spine, the curves in the neck and mid-back should measure between twenty and forty degrees, while the curves in the lower back should be between forty and sixty degrees. Without adequate curvature, the spine is in a weakened position, which will cause it to break down sooner and make it more prone to injury and degeneration over time.

Now let me share with you more details about each of the regions of the spine:

Doctor's Note

Heads up: this section contains quite a few technical and medical terms, so read on to brush up on your body and spine knowledge, or skip to page 57.

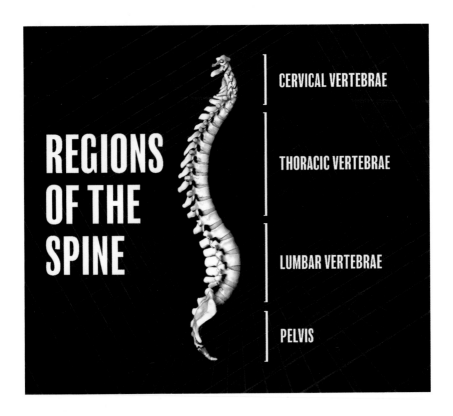

REGIONS OF THE SPINE

CERVICAL VERTEBRAE

THORACIC VERTEBRAE

LUMBAR VERTEBRAE

PELVIS

Cervical spine. The cervical spine, or neck, is the uppermost portion of your spine. In this region, there are seven vertebrae, numbered C1 to C7 from top to bottom. The first two vertebrae in the neck, C1 and C2, are specialized to allow for upper neck and head movement. C1 is called the "atlas," as in Atlas, the Greek god, holding up the world. C1 cradles the skull. C2, called the "axis," has a small bony projection that fits into the atlas, which allows for upper-neck rotation. This is a particularly important neurological area of the spine, because the brain stem, the lowest part of the brain, can be affected by it.

Thoracic spine. There are twelve vertebrae, numbered T1 to T12, in the thoracic part of the spine, also known as the mid-back. The ribs attach to the thoracic part of your spine. The ribs protect your vital organs and, like the vertebrae, have muscles attached to them. This region of your spine is very important for movement of your torso as well as your upper limbs.

Lumbar spine. The lumbar spine, or lower back, consists of five vertebrae, numbered L1 through L5. While some people can have six vertebrae in this region, that is usually a rare occurrence and the result of a genetic "choice," as I call it. The extra vertebra may predispose someone to back pain just because there's more mechanical stress. The lumbar spine connects the thoracic spine to the pelvis. Since the lumbar spine bears the bulk of the body's weight, the vertebrae in this region are the largest.

Pelvis. The pelvis is the lowest part of the spine and consists of the sacrum and the ilium. The sacrum, more commonly known as the tailbone, consists of several vertebrae that fuse together during a baby's development in the womb. The sacrum forms the base of the spine and the backside of your pelvis. The very tip of the sacrum is called the "coccyx." It is a specialized bone where the spinal cord eventually anchors. When you fall on your "tailbone," that bony point is what you land on. It is filled with nerves, which explains why it hurts so much when you land on it.

A CLOSER LOOK AT THE BONES

Now let's get a little closer and look at what comprises each bone or vertebra.

The **body** is the front portion of the bone. Usually box shaped, it is the main weight-bearing structure of the vertebrae.

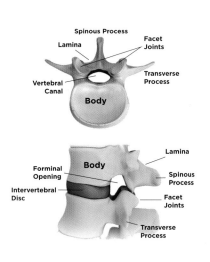

The **spinous process** is the posterior-most (furthest behind) part of the vertebrae. It serves primarily for muscle attachment, and it's the part you can see and feel down someone's back.

The **pedicles** are short, stout, strong parts of the bone that project backwards off the body.

The **lamina** consists of two small plates of bone that join the back of the bone between the pedicles and the spinous process. The function of the lamina is to protect the back part of the spinal cord and the spinal nerves.

The **transverse process** is a bony projection on either side of the vertebrae where the lamina and pedicles join. These are very important for muscle and ligament attachment.

Facet joints are the joints of the spine where one vertebra connects to the vertebra above and below it. These are synovial joints, which means they are enclosed in a ligament sack that contains synovial fluid for lubrication. Where the two opposing surfaces touch, each is covered with cartilage, similar to your knee or other joints of your body. Without healthy joints in your spine, the vertebrae cannot move properly. These are the joints that allow your body to twist and to bend backward and forward and from side to side.

The vertebral canal. All these different bony parts connect to one another, forming a ring with a large opening in the center. This opening is the vertebral canal, through which the spinal cord passes through.

Foraminal openings. Much like the vertebral canal, the neuro-foraminal opening is an opening on either side of the vertebrae that is formed by the articulation or joining of the two adjacent bones. Through this opening exists the thirty-one pairs of spinal nerves, one pair on each side. The foraminal openings are the sites where most nerves get pinched, compressed, or entrapped. When the vertebrae misalign, a condition called "subluxation," the nerve roots can be "pinched" by the bones as they twist and close the opening.

The intervertebral disc. Between each of the vertebrae is a round, cushion-like pad known as an intervertebral disc. These discs are generally symmetrical and have several important functions, including acting as shock absorbers and allowing for normal vertebral range of motion. They act as a pivot point for the bones to roll around, and as a "spacer" between the vertebrae. This space is very important, because it allows the neuroforaminal opening, where the nerve comes out, to be as open as possible.

Discs are filled with a soft, gel-like center called the "nucleus pulposus." This gel center is surrounded by a very strong, fibrous outer layer called the "annulus." Imagine a radial car tire lying flat on the ground with the center of the tire filled with a shock-absorbing jelly. That's similar to the discs that separate and cushion the vertebrae in your spine.

The outer layers of the disc can be damaged by trauma, repetitive movements, or subluxation (dislocation). Since the vertebrae cannot move around, any kind of damage puts constant pressure on the disc. Over time, the annulus (outer layer) can form micro fractures or breaks that allow the gel to push through and form a bulge. This bulge can compress the nerve roots inside the neuroforamen (the hole that it exists in) or the spinal cord. If it gets very serious, it can become a herniation.[29]

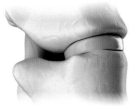
Vertebral Disc

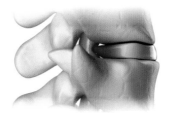
Bulging Vertebral Disc

If the disc material detaches, it is called a "sequestered disc" or "prolapsed disc." That condition is severe and requires surgical intervention. However, with a bulging disc, there are many nonsurgical options for treatment, and these should be used before pursuing surgery, since there is a high failure rate with surgery and often complications arise afterward.

---

29   Author's note: The vast majority of patients who are diagnosed with herniated discs don't have a true herniation, but a bulging disc. Herniations are the most severe form of a bulge, where the protrusion is very large, but it's still intact.

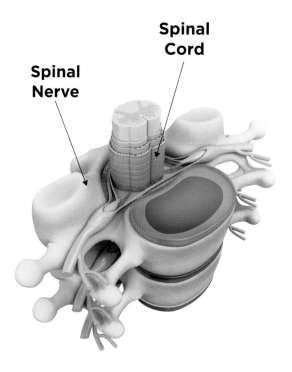

Spinal Nerve

Spinal Cord

THE SPINAL NERVES

As the spinal cord runs down through the vertebral canal, it branches off to form spinal nerves. These nerves are direct extensions of the spinal cord and are part of the central nervous system. They carry direct messages from the brain to all parts of the body, including organs, glands, muscles, and so on, controlling all movement and bodily function.

The spinal nerves branch into thirty-one pairs. These thirty-one pairs of nerves then branch out to form all the millions of nerves in your entire body. Of the thirty-one pairs, eight are found in the neck or cervical spine, twelve are in the mid-back or thoracic spine, and five are in the lower back or lumbar spine. The remaining six pairs are in your sacrum and coccyx. The nerves in the cervical spine control all the structures and organs of the upper chest and arms. The nerves in the thoracic spine control the organs of the chest and abdomen. The nerves in the lumbar spine control the lower abdominal organs and the legs. Structurally, the nerve roots all along the spine pass through the neuroforamina, those openings in the vertebrae that I mentioned earlier.

The higher up in the spine the nerves are located, the more valuable they are to everything below them. That's why when someone damages the spinal cord at the top, they can be paralyzed from the neck down. But if they damage the nerves at the bottom in the lower back, only the areas of the body below the entry site are affected.

THE SOFT TISSUES

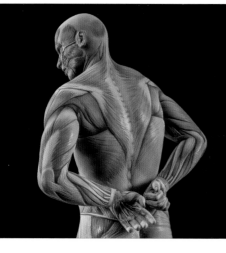

Soft tissues of the back:
- **Muscles**
- **Tendons**
- **Ligaments**

The rest of the "back" is made up of what are called "soft tissues." That includes muscles, tendons, and ligaments. Each of these tissues has a specific purpose.

Muscles are larger structures that provide movement of the body and maintain posture of the body against forces such as gravity. There are large muscle groups that allow for global-type movements, such as walking and turning. Then there are very tiny muscles that are specialized to control fine movements, such as vertebral movement. Some movements are voluntary, meaning you can control them—for instance, raising your arm. Others are involuntary, or reflexes, that can only be controlled by your central nerves.

The tiny muscles have such an important job that your brain doesn't want to leave you in control of. Your brain will let you walk, run, and jump. But allow you to control the fine movements of the vertebrae (the reflexes) that protect your spinal cord and nerves? No way.

Tendons are structures that attach the muscles into the bones to anchor them. The way your body moves is by muscles contracting and pulling on tendons anchored into the bones, causing the bones to move.

Ligaments are very strong bundles of fibers that make a joint stable and strong by holding the bones together. They don't have a lot of give, so they can limit movement of the bone in certain directions to prevent injury.

NOW YOU KNOW

What everyone loosely refers to as their "back" is actually a complex part of the body known as the spine. Calling it the "back" can limit our understanding of how intricate and important the spine is.

By not knowing more about your spine, you may also inadvertently give up control to a doctor who might make a wrong diagnosis or have an agenda in mind when treating you.

Remember Jason, at the beginning of this chapter? Once we determined that the problem was the sacroiliac joint in his pelvis, we treated him with chiropractic adjustments, physical therapy, and acupuncture. Within four weeks, he was free of pain, and within six weeks, he was running again. What do you think would have happened to him if he had followed the recommendations of the orthopedic surgeon and had a double hip replacement?

The spine has one of the most important jobs in the body: to protect the central nervous system, which controls the health and function of every organ, gland, system, and muscle.

When your back or spine is damaged, it can affect multiple other organs, tissues, and systems. Problems with the spine and nerves can be linked to many disorders, such as headaches, TMJ, tinnitus, carpal tunnel syndrome, hip pain, knee pain, neuropathy, and many others. Therefore, knowing about it in more detail, where the pain is coming from, and what to do about it is paramount. In the coming chapters, we will cover those important points.

TAKE IT ←··OR··→ LEAVE IT

- You only get one chance to have a healthy spine. Choose wisely how you care for it.

- Without a basic understanding of your spine, you can't make the best decisions for your care. You will essentially give over control to a doctor who may be wrong or may have another motive.

- A healthy spine isn't just about a healthy column of bones and discs. The vital nerves that branch off the spinal cord control everything in your body: muscles, heart, lungs, immune system, and so on.

- To be healthy, all these individual structures must work together. Problems with one create problems with the others. Therefore, treating multiple structures or tissues is the best solution.

Visit drbradfordbutler.com for more information.

- @dr_bbutler
- www.facebook.com/drbradfordbutler
- www.linkedin.com/in/dr-brad-butler

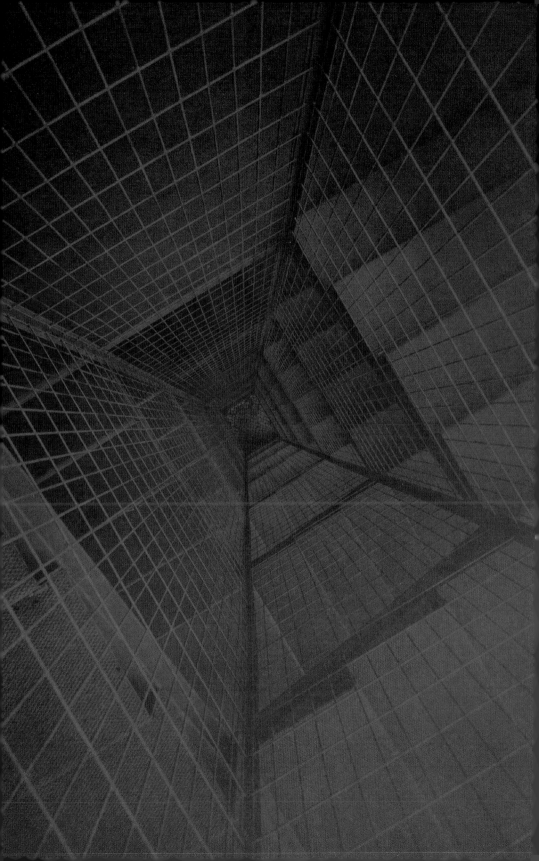

CHAPTER FIVE

DECONSTRUCTING BACK PAIN— KNOWING WHAT TO TREAT

My experience over the years has proven to me that the typical path a patient chooses for his or her back or neck pain is *not* the one that you want to take.

As I stated in an earlier chapter, what is considered the "traditional" or "conventional" approach is the least successful. Why people continue to follow that approach has a lot to do with marketing—both inside and outside of the medical profession—that intentionally influences by disparaging non-drug therapies that do work or by promoting new drugs or even old ones using falsified or suspicious data.

The June 2017 issue of *Consumer Reports* magazine was dedicated to "Real Relief from Back Pain." In the issue, Donald Levy, MD, states that conventional treatment fails because "it focuses on individual symptoms and broken parts."[30] In other words, if you're going

---

30 Teresa Carr, "The Better Way to Get Back Pain Relief," *Consumer Reports*, May 4, 2017, accessed August 19, 2017, https://www.consumerreports.org/back-pain/the-better-way-to-get-back-pain-relief/.

to your family doctor wanting to fix what's wrong with your back, you're going to the wrong place. That's because his or her focus is on just one component of the problem, such as pain. Or he or she is looking for one single cause of the pain and treating that one cause. Further, traditional or conventional medical training is generally geared toward treating the symptom of back pain, viewing that *symptom* as the problem. It is not focused on treating the problem, which is *causing* the symptoms.

ALEXIS: THE PROBLEM WASN'T HER WRISTS

When Alexis came to see me, she had already undergone surgery for carpal tunnel in both wrists. Unfortunately, the surgery didn't resolve her pain and strength issues, so she continued to suffer for years. I examined her and discovered that the pain in her wrists and hands was coming from nerves compressed in her neck. We treated her neck, and her wrist pain went away—we never even treated her wrists.

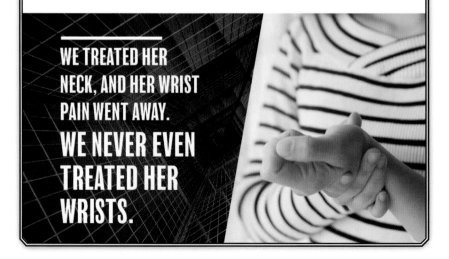

WE TREATED HER NECK, AND HER WRIST PAIN WENT AWAY. WE NEVER EVEN TREATED HER WRISTS.

Now, you might think that a traditional doctor could use science and tests to prove what's causing the pain and then prescribe an effective treatment. But again, you'd be wrong. Sure, they may do some tests, but the results of these tests lead them to the same treatment: drug therapy.

In fact, the *Consumer Reports* article, which is based on research from a 2013 *Journal of the American Medical Association* (JAMA) study, found that the more studies doctors ordered, the more prescriptions they wrote.

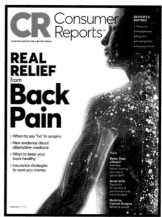

The JAMA study correlated that there was a specific relationship between increased visual studies, like MRI and CT scans, and significantly increased rates of powerful prescription drugs prescribed.

Richard Deyo, MD, author and professor, was quoted as saying, "These kinds of escalating interventions are still the hallmark of how back pain is usually treated in the U.S.," and that "overall, we've seen no reduction in pain or disability"[31] because of conventional approaches.

Deyo also said that "conventional approaches don't always work and can cause other serious problems." Instead, Levy said, those of us in the medical profession who are treating patients "should be thinking about treating *the whole* patient" (emphasis added). [32]

Essentially, the doctors in the *Consumer Reports* expose were saying that patients can be duped because their doctor may use

---

31 Teresa Carr, "The Better Way to Get Back Pain Relief," *Consumer Reports*, May 4, 2017, accessed August 19, 2017, https://www.consumerreports.org/back-pain/the-better-way-to-get-back-pain-relief/.

32 Ibid.

impressive technology to "show" them where the pain is coming from, but they still get prescription drugs as treatment. And some of those prescriptions are very powerful and have dangerous side effects. Plus, the use of technology hasn't even made a difference in their success rates.

The rest of this chapter is designed to give you the whole story so that you can treat the whole problem and not get lost in the quagmire of chasing symptoms through drugs and surgery.

First let me review some basic points from the last chapter.

ESSENTIALLY, THE DOCTORS IN THE *CONSUMER REPORTS* EXPOSE WERE SAYING THAT PATIENTS CAN BE DUPED, BECAUSE THEIR DOCTOR MAY USE IMPRESSIVE TECHNOLOGY TO "SHOW" THEM WHERE THE PAIN IS COMING FROM, BUT THEY STILL GET PRESCRIPTION DRUGS AS TREATMENT.

- Your spine is a very important structure made up of multiple parts and tissues.

- The primary functions of your spine are to protect the incredibly important spinal cord and spinal nerves, which control all body functions and movements.

- The spine is also designed to support your body weight and allow you to move.

Remember: When you are talking about your back, you are really talking about your spine.

Also take a moment to recall what I discussed earlier in the book: Patients are not concerned only with the pain they're experiencing, even though that seems to be top of mind. The real reason they want to be pain-free is to be able to do the things that the pain has stopped them from doing. The loss of function due to the pain—that's their real concern. Without your spine, you can't stand, keep yourself upright, move about freely, bend, or have flexibility. In other words, when you have moderate or severe back pain, all the things your spine is supposed to do when it's healthy and working properly, you can't do. You simply can't function in life: You can't get in and out of the car with ease, you can't clean your house, and forget about lifting or carrying anything. Forget about being active.

But is it just the bones that are causing the problem? No. While the pain and disability can come from the vertebrae, it can

WITHOUT YOUR SPINE, YOU CAN'T STAND, KEEP YOURSELF UPRIGHT, MOVE ABOUT FREELY, BEND, OR HAVE FLEXIBILITY. IN OTHER WORDS, WHEN YOU HAVE MODERATE OR SEVERE BACK PAIN, ALL THE THINGS YOUR SPINE IS SUPPOSED TO DO WHEN IT'S HEALTHY AND WORKING PROPERLY, YOU CAN'T DO.

also come from any or all the following: joints, muscles, ligaments, discs, nerves, or inflammation of any of these structures. When you have damage to one or more of these structures, you will get pain.

In my experience, damage is usually present with several at the same time. That is why knowing the cause of the pain is so important. Can you treat a muscle the same way you treat a nerve? Can you treat a nerve the same way you treat a joint? Can you treat a joint the same way as a disc? The answer to all of these is *no*.

TWO KINDS OF DAMAGE—INJURIES AND DEGENERATION

To give you a better idea of what I'm talking about with damage, let's look at what is called a "spinal motion segment."

A motion segment refers to two adjacent vertebrae and the connecting tissue that binds them together. The five physical structures that lead to pain are nerves, joints, discs, muscles, and ligaments.

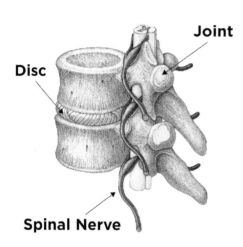

Disc • **Joint** • **Spinal Nerve**

Motion Segment
(not shown: muscles and ligaments)

A sixth cause, inflammation, can happen if any of these structures get damaged or irritated. Damage can occur when these structures become injured or—and this is important—after long periods of breakdown or degeneration.

Keep in mind, especially with degeneration, that more than one area is usually involved in the pain. How does it happen that multiple areas get involved? Well, first let me discuss injuries.

Injuries are easy to explain. They usually happen in one of two ways: trauma or overuse.

A traumatic injury is an injury that can occur with a "sudden onset," such as a sports injury, fall, car accident, or an activity of daily living that causes sudden damage, such as lifting something that's too heavy or lifting the wrong way or just moving in an unnatural way.

An overuse injury is one that typically happens with a repetitive movement over time. The Mayo Clinic defines it as "any type of muscle or joint injury, such as tendonitis or a stress fracture, that's caused by repetitive trauma." It states that an overuse injury usually stems from training errors, which can occur when a person takes on too much physical activity too quickly.[33]

While I find that definition to be useful, I don't feel it applies to the average person. Instead, I define an overuse injury as something that happens when someone does the same movement patterns over and over for such a period of time that it leads to damage to one or more tissues.

For example, if you're a plumber, you are constantly putting yourself in an awkward position that can create mechanical disadvantages for your back. When you are in these positions, you are often straining by lifting, pushing, pulling, twisting, and turning, which can lead to micro-

> **I DEFINE AN OVERUSE INJURY AS SOMETHING THAT HAPPENS WHEN SOMEONE DOES THE SAME MOVEMENT PATTERNS OVER AND OVER FOR SUCH A PERIOD OF TIME THAT IT LEADS TO DAMAGE TO ONE OR MORE TISSUES.**

traumas to the tissues in your spine. These microtraumas accumulate over time, until one day you cross the threshold where there is too much damage, and then it's as if "suddenly" you hurt your back.

The same can be said for any profession where a person does the same things day in and day out, such as hairstylists, electricians, cooks, computer workers, driving professionals, landscapers, and even doctors and nurses. A sedentary lifestyle in which a person stays

---

33   "Overuse injury: How to prevent training injuries," Mayo Clinic, accessed August 19, 2017, http://www.mayoclinic.org/healthy-lifestyle/fitness/in-depth/overuse-injury/art-20045875.

in the same position for long periods of time can also lead to an overuse injury.

So, while overuse can happen with training, in my experience, patients who create small amounts of damage over a long period of time, resulting in an overuse injury, concern me the most.

WHY? BECAUSE WHEN YOU ARE DEVELOPING INJURIES OR DAMAGE OVER MANY YEARS, THE SYMPTOMS CAN BE LESS SEVERE OR DON'T LAST AS LONG AS A "SUDDEN ONSET" OF A TRAUMA.

Why? Because when you are developing injuries or damage over many years, the symptoms can be less severe or don't last as long as a "sudden onset" of a trauma. As a result, you can be lulled into a false sense that your problem is minor, and you may not take it seriously.

For many people, months or even years can go by before they are forced to address a problem they've been having. During that time, the injury is getting more and more severe.

As I discussed in earlier chapters, time can be your best friend or it can be your biggest enemy. Let's look at how time makes things worse.

THE PHASES OF DEGENERATION

The diagram adjacent is essentially a time-lapse representation of what will happen to your back, neck, or spine problem over time if it is not corrected. Much like tooth decay, degeneration of the parts of the spine I detailed earlier in the chapter, when left untreated, will go from mild to moderate to severe.

STAGES OF DEGENERATION

1

1-20 YEARS OLD
REQUIRES 4-8 WEEKS OF CARE

CHIROPRACTIC
NEUROMUSCULAR RE-EDUCATION

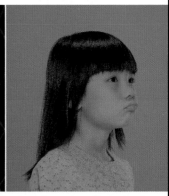

2

21-40 YEARS OLD
REQUIRES 8-12 WEEKS OF CARE

CHIROPRACTIC
NEUROMUSCULAR REEDUCATION
PHYSICAL THERAPY
ACUPUNCTURE

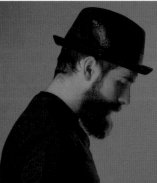

3

41-60 YEARS OLD
REQUIRES 8-12 WEEKS OF CARE

CHIROPRACTIC
NEUROMUSCULAR RE-EDUCATION
PHYSICAL THERAPY   LASER THERAPY
ACUPUNCTURE   DECOMPRESSION
MASSAGE

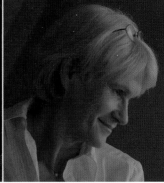

4

60+ YEARS OLD
REQUIRES 12+ WEEKS OF CARE

CHIROPRACTIC
NEUROMUSCULAR RE-EDUCATION
PHYSICAL THERAPY   LASER THERAPY
ACUPUNCTURE   DECOMPRESSION
MASSAGE

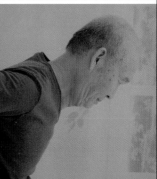

Problems or injuries to one structure will spread to other structures. That happens because an injury to one tissue can force another structure or tissue to overcompensate. Essentially, that means the other structure or tissue gets overstressed and overworked, which leads to it also breaking down at an accelerated rate. It becomes a downward spiral.

As an example, a very common problem in the spine is called a "subluxation." A subluxation is when a vertebra gets "stuck" out of its normal position due to a variety of reasons: an injury, bad posture, repetitive movements, and so forth. The joints become locked, much like a link in a chain can get turned a certain way and become locked up.

The subluxation in and of itself may not cause any pain, but because the joints must move to help take stress off the vertebrae and the discs, if the joints lock, the weight of the body can become stuck on the discs. Without normal vertebral motion to keep the disc healthy, it will begin to lose water content over many years, a condition called "desiccation."

As the disc continues to lose fluid, it becomes weaker and weaker. That weakening can allow the gel that makes up the center of the disc to start to fracture. Eventually, the outer layer of the disc can't contain the gel and a bulge is created. This bulge can then press on the spinal nerve and cause severe pain.

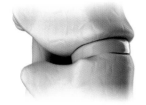
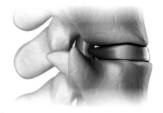
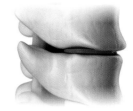

Vertebral Disc   Bulging Vertebral Disc   Degenerated Vertebral Disc

That raises several questions: What was the cause—the disc pressing on the nerve, or the joints being locked out of position (subluxation)? Also, if you just treat the disc via drugs or surgery and don't address the joint problems, what will happen over time? Well, the answer to the latter question is this: since the cause was never truly fixed, the procedure will eventually fail and the problem will return.

That's what happened to Michaela, a young mother who came to see me several years ago. She was only twenty-seven at the time, but she had suffered from debilitating migraines since she was a young teen. Michaela told me that the pain from headaches was so bad that it was impossible to get through the day. She felt like she was a terrible mom, because the pain kept her from being able to be the caring mother she wanted to be with her young child. Her pain was severely affecting her life.

About ten years earlier at the age of around seventeen, she had also started to develop pain in her neck and upper back. She never connected the pain in her neck and upper back with her headaches, even though they were in fact linked. Why? Because her mother, following "conventional" thought, took her to the family doctor,

> **IF YOU JUST TREAT THE DISC VIA DRUGS OR SURGERY AND DON'T ADDRESS THE JOINT PROBLEMS, WHAT WILL HAPPEN OVER TIME? WELL, THE ANSWER TO THE LATTER QUESTION IS THIS: SINCE THE CAUSE WAS NEVER TRULY FIXED, THE PROCEDURE WILL EVENTUALLY FAIL AND THE PROBLEM WILL RETURN.**

who diagnosed her with headaches, and yes, gave her a prescription for headache medicine.

After years of the medicine being ineffective—yes, years of a teenager suffering—Michaela was finally referred to a neurologist, who ran a series of tests and then prescribed an even stronger migraine medication. In the end, the diagnosis was based purely on Michaela's symptomatic presentation (pain at the base of the skull spreading to behind her eyes that was so severe it created visual auras) and no evidence.

So, at the old age of twenty-seven, Michaela came to see me—not because of her headaches, but because of the increase in severe neck pain that radiated to her upper back and shoulders. My team and I performed a comprehensive evaluation and took X-rays of her neck. What shocked us all was that, at twenty-seven, a part of Michaela's neck looked like it belonged to someone in their seventies. At the C5/C6 level, there was almost no disc space remaining, which meant that the disc had deteriorated by over 80 percent—and she was only twenty-seven!

The bones adjacent to that disc also showed signs of advanced decay. The most interesting thing, though, was that above and below that specific area, all the other vertebrae and discs were normal. There was no sign of decay at all.

As a doctor, that meant one thing to me. There must have been a trauma to her head or neck, but that extent of damage takes at least twenty years to develop. That meant something happened when she was a child, but she had reported no history of injury or trauma.

So, I met with Michaela and told her my findings. Surprisingly, she denied ever having had any injury or trauma. I maintained my position and told her to go home and ask her mother if she remembered anything that could have caused an injury.

Sure enough, when Michaela came back for her treatment the next day, she reported that her mother told her about a car accident the two of them had been in when Michaela was three years old. They were involved in a head-on collision, and Michaela was launched from the backseat of the car over the front seat and into the windshield, hitting it with her head—this was before there were seatbelt laws. Of course, Michaela cried hysterically for several minutes while her terrified mother cradled her, but in the end, her mother said, she seemed okay. She had a bad bump on her head, but it wasn't bleeding. And she had some torticollis, or neck stiffness, for a few days. But since all the symptoms eventually subsided, Michaela was never even taken to the doctor. Bingo! Twenty-four years later, she was now in my office.

My team and I began an integrated system of care with Michaela. Since twenty-four years had passed since the trauma, it took her several weeks before her body began to respond. Around six weeks in, Michaela came in with no neck pain. She also reported that the migraines she had experienced and been heavily medicated for as a youth were noticeably less severe. Finally, after just twelve weeks, Michaela was pain-free; she had no more migraines, no more neck pain, and no more upper-back pain.

The program we put her on

AFTER JUST TWELVE WEEKS OF THE RIGHT KIND OF CARE, WE WERE ABLE TO REVERSE TWENTY-FOUR YEARS OF DAMAGE.

addressed all the causes of her pain: the joints, nerves, discs, muscles, and ligaments. After just twelve weeks of the right kind of care, we were able to reverse twenty-four years of damage. Michaela was able to get through the day without pain for the first time since she was a child. She was happier in general, and she felt so much better as a mother because she now had the energy to be able to be present with her child.

After her treatment, Michaela remarked that she had forgotten what it was like to be normal. She had thought she was going to have to live with pain for the rest of her life.

Michaela's story isn't just an isolated "miracle." Her story is one of thousands of stories of patients who have recovered when they thought all hope was lost.

When treatment involves all the components at the same time, the body can finally heal and regain function.

What may be most surprising to you are the non-spine symptoms that frequently originate in the spine. In fact, we have successfully helped hundreds of patients like Michaela, who never even knew her misdiagnosed migraines were originating in her neck. We have helped patients alleviate pain in other areas of the body that is originating from the spine, including headaches and pain in the jaw, hips, knees, shoulders, wrists, hands, feet, and more.

We can even help when medical interventions or surgeries don't resolve pain and discomfort. One reason procedures often don't work is that the doctor or surgeon treats the location of the pain and not the location of the real problem. When you treat the source of the problem, the results can be far reaching.

TAKE IT ←···OR···→ LEAVE IT

- Know something about your back so that you can make smarter choices.

- Your back is not just one thing. It is many structures. Each of these structures can be the cause of your pain, but usually it's more than one. Knowing which non-drug, nonsurgical therapies are most effective will be the focus of the rest of this book.

- Focusing on the symptoms may not indicate where the actual source of your pain is.

- More tests by your doctor doesn't equal better results.

- You don't hurt your back only through trauma. Overuse and repetition can do just as much damage over time and may be more dangerous because you are more likely to mask the symptoms.

- Problems with your spine can cause other problems away from the spine. These can include problems with your head, neck, shoulders, arms, hands, hips, knees, and feet, just to name a few.

Visit drbradfordbutler.com for more information.

ⓨ @dr_bbutler

ⓕ www.facebook.com/drbradfordbutler

ⓘ www.linkedin.com/in/dr-brad-butler

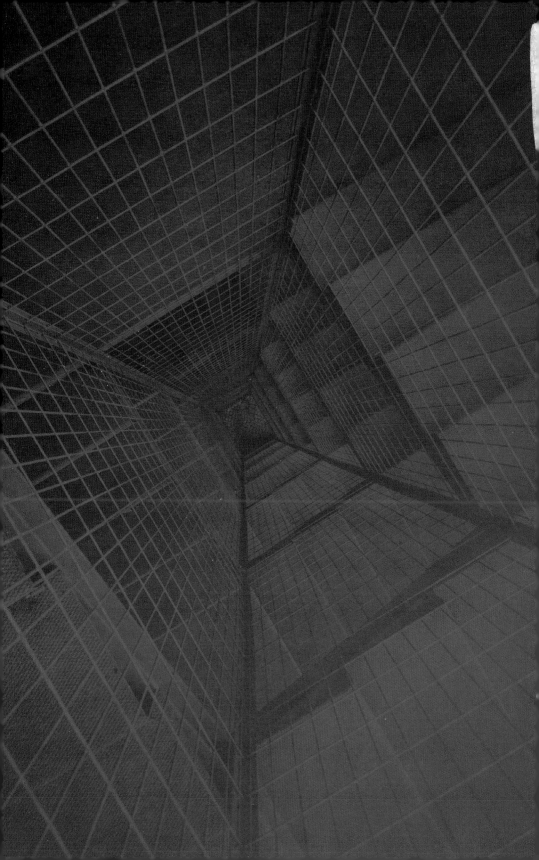

CHAPTER SIX

SETTING A GOAL VS. EXCUSES, DRUGS, SURGERY

A goal properly set is halfway reached.

—*Zig Ziglar*

Before you can *achieve* what you want, you have to know what it is you are shooting for. It's surprising how many people are great at complaining about something, but when you ask them what they truly want, they can't accurately and specifically identify it. You know who I'm talking about. It might be someone you hear repeatedly say, "I have to lose weight." But that statement is so vague that it's not surprising that they never actually get around to taking any weight off.

If you really want to achieve something, you must be specific about it. Losing weight, for instance, would be a lot more achievable with a statement such as "I want to weigh 180 pounds by Thanksgiving, and to do that I'm going to do X, Y, and Z."

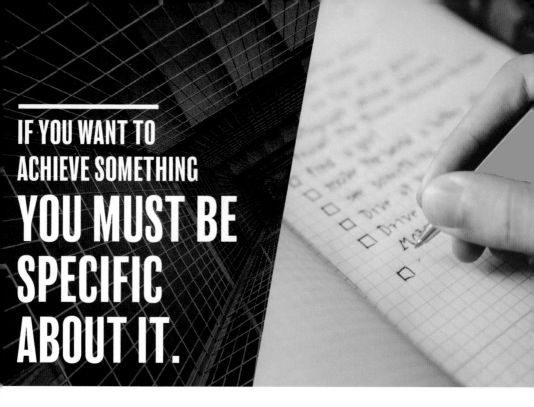

IF YOU WANT TO ACHIEVE SOMETHING YOU MUST BE SPECIFIC ABOUT IT.

The rest of this book will mean nothing to you if you don't have specific goals. In the pages ahead, you will be given a plan to feel great again along with the evidence that you *can* feel great again. If your goal is to live a longer, healthier, pain-free life, then continue reading. If, however, you are reading this book just to cheat the system, if you are looking for yet another shortcut to pain relief no matter the future consequences, then you should stop reading now and go back to drugs and surgery.

When I speak at seminars or to large groups about back pain, I am very honest. I tell the audience that having a goal of "just feeling good" is a fool's game. There are lots of ways to feel good by taking drugs—both legal and illegal, by the way—but none of them will fix the problem.

This chapter will focus on goals and inspiration. I will use some of my favorite quotes to signify the importance of goals and how to achieve them. These quotes will help you stay on course and navigate your way so that you don't get trapped in the swamp that is the current health care cartel between the drug companies, the hospitals, and the government, which have aligned against your goals in the name of profits. Ready? Here are my favorite goal-setting quotes:

YOU GET WHAT YOU DESERVE. ~ JAY GEIER

I remember the first time my consultant shared this quote with a group I was in. My initial reaction was one of anger and frustration, much like yours might be right now. "What do you mean I get what I deserve? It's not my fault I have severe back pain," you might be saying.

To put this quote into context, Jay was talking to a group of about a hundred doctors, not about back pain, but about the pain they all had from their struggling practices. But what he was saying about their "practice health" pertains to you and your back health.

See, in the world of health care, there are some doctors who are very successful, and there are others who severely struggle to be successful. The ones who succeed have certain things in common, as do the ones who are failing. I'll discuss what those who are succeeding have in common in the next chapter, *Healing by Design*.

WHEN I SPEAK AT SEMINARS OR TO LARGE GROUPS ABOUT BACK PAIN, I AM VERY HONEST. I TELL THE AUDIENCE THAT HAVING A GOAL OF "JUST FEELING GOOD" IS A FOOL'S GAME. THERE ARE LOTS OF WAYS TO FEEL GOOD BY TAKING DRUGS—BOTH LEGAL AND ILLEGAL, BY THE WAY—BUT NONE OF THEM WILL FIX THE PROBLEM.

Over the years, I've counseled many, many doctors in various fields. The ones who struggle share the same weaknesses, which is why they all suffer.

So, what are these common traits? First, they have no clearly defined goals. Second, they don't have a specific written plan to achieve them. Third, they don't have objective—not subjective—metrics that will tell them whether they are progressing. Fourth, they're always looking for the magic bullet or the quick fix. And finally, fifth, they're filled with excuses as to why things are different about their situation. Kind of amazing, right?

Well, I see the exact same thing from chronic back pain sufferers. The ways they attempt to accomplish their ill-defined goal to "get out of pain" include:

- Having no specific plan to accomplish their goal.

- Jumping from doctor to doctor, from therapy to therapy, and from drug to drug.

- Having no objective way of measuring their progress. They base everything only on how they feel, which is imperfect at best, because lots of things can affect how you feel.

- Barely giving anything time to work and then moving on to the next magic bullet (procedure, potion, or lotion, as we refer to it in the industry).

And they tell me all the "reasons" they can't get better:

- "It runs in my family."
- "I tried everything and nothing works."
- "I was diagnosed with X [insert any diagnosis you want]."
- "My doctor said surgery is the only thing that will work."

These excuses are the same types of things I hear from the failing doctors I speak with. You hear all of the excuses as to why he or she isn't succeeding, things like "I live in a bad town," or "I don't have good insurance in my area like you do," or "You must get good patients. I don't get good patients in my area." The list of excuses goes on and on.

So, what's the point? Just like the failing doctor, the failing back pain patient spends all their time complaining about their problem and *justifying* why nothing will work for them. They always want to blame others for their lack of success. They don't want to be accountable or responsible for their actions.

But just as I proved earlier in this book, *you don't have that luxury anymore*. You are now at a point where it's "fix it or else."

> **OUR CORE BELIEF IS "OVER DELIVERING" FOR OUR PATIENTS. OVER DELIVERING FOR PATIENTS MEANS CREATING A "WOW" EXPERIENCE LIKE THEY NEVER HAD AT A DOCTOR'S OFFICE BEFORE.**

People who are unsuccessful at anything, in my experience, put more energy into why something isn't working than on new solutions to make it work. They like to blame outside factors, things that they have no control over and therefore have no responsibility for. Are you one of those people? Are you someone who puts more energy and focus into why you can't be successful than into doing the things that will make you successful?

One key factor that has made my practices some of the most successful in the country and the reason we have plans to open more than twenty additional locations in the next five years is our core belief in "over delivering" for our patients. Over delivering for patients means creating a "wow" experience like they've never had at a doctor's office before. They leave after every treatment feeling as if they just had the best experience they've ever had in a doctor's office. Why? Because that was the specific goal I had when I opened my first practice twenty years ago. And because I have a specific plan for patients that is based around over delivering, I expected that result.

Because we over deliver, our patients are compelled to share their stories with their friends and family members. And they refer patients to us who truly want the best experience in the best environment, with the best providers and staff. So even though one of our practices is in the small town of Oakland, New Jersey, in an average location, it provides more care for more people than the vast majority of offices in the country. In fact, people drive for miles and miles, passing untold numbers of competitors, to get to this office.

Why? Because we don't buy into excuses of what can't be done, but focus on the goal "to help as many people as possible live a longer, healthier, happier, pain-free life." We do that with a specific plan to over deliver in every area, on every visit. We don't give any attention to excuses like small towns or mediocre location. Instead, we built the most beautiful office we could in that ordinary location and filled it with the best, most highly trained providers and staff.

When I hear doctors struggling and complaining, I tell them, "You get what you deserve." Why? Because they put very little attention into the patient's wants and needs. They're open during hours that are only convenient for them and their lifestyles, but very inconvenient for a patient. As a result, they make patients wait on every visit before they see the doctor while we, on the other hand, have a no-waiting policy. They make it difficult for new patients to make appointments in a reasonable amount of time and often make them wait for weeks or even months, while we have a same-day guarantee.

They often limit health services because that's what makes them feel comfortable. We have a vision of "everything under one roof," so the patient can see multiple providers on the same appointment in the same location for their convenience. They have a total focus on insurance as the payor. We offer affordable plans for the uninsured or underinsured.

In other words, their offices are designed for *their* needs and wants, and ours are designed for what a *patient* who really wants to get better would need and want.

I have a question for you. Which of the aforementioned offices is easier and cheaper to set up and run? If you guessed the unsuccessful doctor, you'd be right. To create insanely successful practices, like I have, all the hard work is done up front, and the success comes after lots of trial and error, lots of sweat and tears, lots of learning from frustrations—and it takes time!

The industrialist Andrew Carnegie said: "If you want to be happy, set a goal that commands your thoughts, liberates your energy, and inspires your hope." You see, to achieve something of value, it takes your thought, your energy, your efforts, and your inspiration—with hope that you'll achieve it. Nothing of value, like your health, can be achieved using the cheapest method, the fastest method, or the easiest method.

The reason I share this example of the successful versus the unsuccessful doctor is that there is a similarity between what it takes to heal and what it takes to be successful. If your goal is to cut corners with your back or look for the quick fix, an easier solution, then don't be surprised if you "get what you deserve."

ALL WHO HAVE ACCOMPLISHED GREAT THINGS HAVE HAD A GREAT AIM, HAVE FIXED THEIR GAZE ON A GOAL WHICH WAS HIGH, ONE WHICH SOMETIMES SEEMED IMPOSSIBLE. ~ ORISON SWETT MARDEN

The problem I have seen over the last twenty years is that things are getting worse and not better with patients. Many industries evolve as time moves on. They create new paradigms that lead to more success. We've seen it in computers, printers, cell phones, sharing of information, automobiles, how we shop, investing—the list goes on and on.

But with back and neck pain, it's just the opposite. Not much has changed over twenty years. Sure, there are new "drugs" that hit the market, but in time they prove they aren't any better than the old ones. There are new procedures, like laser surgery, but it's just a new spin, using a new gadget.

What is consistent is that what you are being sold is hype over results. It's called "the shiny new object syndrome," where because something is new, we assume it's better and gets better results. For example: Is that stupid pillow that guy sells on TV really *the best pillow ever made*? Or is it just a new spin and he's selling us all on a sensational idea? (Doctor's note: Don't waste your money. A lot of my patients bought them as their solution—or should I say "quick fix to neck pain"—and then threw them out.)

IF YOU DON'T KNOW WHERE YOU'RE GOING, ANY ROAD WILL GET YOU THERE. ~ LEWIS CARROLL

If you don't even know what your real goal is, then how can you ever achieve it? You need to be very clear on where you want to be, and where you don't want to be. Mark Twain said, "Whenever you find yourself on the side of the majority, it's time to pause and reflect."

The first part of this book described in detail what the "majority" has and is doing. Now it's time for you to reflect and set new goals.

The problem is, most people don't know how to set goals, specifically for their health. Instead, they feel unempowered with their health, which is exactly what the "cartel" wants you to be. How do you set a goal when it comes to your back and neck pain? It's simple. Goals are things that you want to achieve. Oxford Dictionaries defines a goal as: "The object of a person's ambition or effort; an aim or desired result."

Now, let me ask you a question: When it comes to your back pain, do you have an aim or desired result? Let me ask you another question that pertains to the first part of the definition: Have you been a passive participant and just done what you were told to do, like a sheep, or have you demonstrated ambition and put in the effort to heal?

Effort refers to the time, energy, and investment to get better. Without those three components, you cannot get better.

So, step one in setting a goal is to write it down. An anonymous person once said, "Goals that are not written down are just wishes." You must clarify what you really want so that you can reflect on what it takes to get it. Most patients I meet have no goals for their health, let alone written ones. That is such a shock to me with something as important as their health. As you write down your goals, I think you will be amazed to see that the vast majority of them deal not with feeling better, but with being able to do things again.

Earlier I said that most patients say they want to feel better, but what they really want is to be able to do the things they used to be able to do but can't because of the pain. I bring that up because you will see that if you make a list, things like:

- To sit for more than a few minutes—without pain.

- To sleep better—without pain.

- To be able to walk upstairs—without pain.

- Do yard work—without pain.

- Play with or hold my kids or grandkids—without pain.

- Get out of a chair—without pain.

- Do my job—without pain.

Notice that the first part of everything on the list is an action that a healthy, functioning person can do. You never see the list in reverse. You never see "I want to get rid of my pain so that I can go to work," "I want to get rid of my pain so I can pick up my kids," "I want to get rid of my pain so I can hold my grandkids." It's a significant point I'm making here, because it's totally incongruent with what you are doing for your back and neck. It's totally backwards, right?

Think about it. What if I said to you, "I want to get in shape so that I can go to the gym"? You would look at me funny. Someone who says they want to get in shape first is the kind of person who sits at home and buys things that promise to help them get in shape without doing anything that will get them in shape. They buy vitamins, supplements, weight loss products, DVDs (sounds like a billion-dollar industry to me). On the other hand, someone who says "I need to get to the gym to get in shape" is the kind of person who puts in the time, the energy, and the investment to do what it takes to get in shape.

Again, that's what it takes: time, energy, and investment. And that begins by writing down your goal. Write down what you really want in as much detail as possible. Then we will talk about the plan.

BY RECORDING YOUR DREAMS AND GOALS ON PAPER, YOU SET IN MOTION THE PROCESS OF BECOMING THE PERSON YOU MOST WANT TO BE. PUT YOUR FUTURE IN GOOD HANDS—YOUR OWN. ~ MARK VICTOR HANSEN

I love that quote by Mark Victor Hansen. It truly encompasses everything you need to do. Write it down, set it in motion, be accountable, and over time you will see great things.

Before we get to the plan (in the next chapter), I want to tell you a quick story about an experience I had when I took my daughter Kelsie for a lunch date at our local diner. The waitress sat us down right next to two elderly gentlemen. As many of you know, when two older guys go to lunch, they typically are going to be talking about one of two things, either politics or the latest health crisis they're dealing with. It was impossible for me not to overhear about all the problems, drugs, and injections the one gentleman was getting. Wherever I go, I seem to have bionic ears for people who are suffering and doing the wrong things for their suffering but think they're doing the right things.

> **THAT'S WHAT IT TAKES: TIME, ENERGY, AND INVESTMENT. AND THAT BEGINS BY WRITING DOWN YOUR GOAL. WRITE DOWN WHAT YOU REALLY WANT IN AS MUCH DETAIL AS POSSIBLE. THEN WE WILL TALK ABOUT THE PLAN.**

As Kelsie and I finished up, I looked at her and I said, "Listen, honey, before we go, I have to go over and talk to these two guys in the booth next to you. Please don't be embarrassed." Lucky for me, at thirteen years old, she has watched me do this many, many times. I feel compelled to help people—what can I say?

I grabbed a chair and I pulled it up to the booth where the two were sitting, and said, "Hey guys." As you can imagine, there was an uncomfortable and stunned look on their faces. After introducing myself and telling them what I do for a living, they opened up a little bit. It turns out that the one with all the problems was an eighty-four-year-old retired dentist. Now, as a doctor, he was very interested in how I explained what we do at Oakland Spine & Physical Therapy. And both men were interested when I explained why our method of thinking is the way that *they* should be thinking about most of their problems (pain, radiating pain, numbness and tingling, neuropathy).

I explained to the retired dentist that all he was doing was putting a Band-Aid on the real problems, which were a lack of normal function that led to his symptoms. He asked why the doctors had done everything to him, including—wait for it—surgery on his wrist, that didn't help the neuropathy (numbness and tingling in his hand and fingers). Here again, the approach was backwards. Doctors, I explained, for better or worse, follow what are called "standards of care." That means they must do everything possible that would normally be done medically, even if they don't necessarily think that a patient like him needed it. If they didn't, they could be sued if something went wrong or got worse and an attorney found out that they didn't follow the "standard of care" for this condition.

It sounds crazy, but much of what goes on at the doctor's office is what is referred to in the industry as "CYA (cover-your-ass) medicine." In other words, you might not need something (a drug, shot, test, or procedure), but if the doctor doesn't use "standard of care" treatment, he or she could be found liable. So that's why they do what they do.

The elderly dentist smiled at me and said, "You know, when I first got into dentistry, it was the same thing." He said, "Back then, if you were going to fill a cavity, it was considered a standard of care that you had to wipe down the entire tooth with alcohol. So, we did it even though we knew that the alcohol would cause the tooth to disintegrate and eventually die." I asked him, "When did that standard change?" And he said, "When they finally realized we were killing the same tooth we were trying to help."

Now, if you read the beginning of this book and understood the results of what the "masses" are doing and what's behind those insane standards of care (or CYA treatment options), then maybe you want a better plan.

MUCH OF WHAT GOES ON AT THE DOCTOR'S OFFICE IS WHAT IS REFERRED TO IN THE INDUSTRY AS "CYA (COVER-YOUR-ASS) MEDICINE." IN OTHER WORDS, YOU MIGHT NOT NEED SOMETHING (A DRUG, SHOT, TEST, OR PROCEDURE), BUT IF THE DOCTOR DOESN'T USE "STANDARD OF CARE" TREATMENT, HE OR SHE COULD BE FOUND LIABLE.

In the next chapter, I will go over the best treatment options, why they're the best, and how you should utilize them. I will also review the Butler Spine Program and what makes it so special.

First, however, you must define your goals. I suggest that you bring them to your doctor's office and ask how what he or she is doing is going to get you closer to those goals, instead of just using a Band-Aid.

- *All successful people have a goal. No one can get anywhere unless he knows where he wants to go and what he wants to be or do. ~ Norman Vincent Peale.*

- Without a goal, you lack a compass. You can't get where you want to go unless you define what you really want.

- Goals must be written. The more detailed, the better. These written goals allow you to ask better questions and get more accurate answers.

- Be careful not to blindly follow standards of care. The treatments must make sense, because not all standards of care are in your best interest.

- When it comes to your back, you truly get what you deserve. It might sound like tough love, but it's true. Your decisions determine what you get. Choose wisely!

Visit drbradfordbutler.com for more information.

🐦 **@dr_bbutler**

ⓕ **www.facebook.com/drbradfordbutler**

ⓘ **www.linkedin.com/in/dr-brad-butler**

CHAPTER SEVEN

HEALING BY DESIGN

Goals. There's no telling what you can do when you get
inspired by them. There's no telling what you can do
when you believe in them. There's no telling what will
happen when you **act** *upon them [emphasis added].*

—*Jim Rohn*

O ne of the great things about having a plan is that it lets you
see how the pieces of the puzzle fit together. It allows you to
feel good that you have a system to follow, and it allows you
to have more faith because what you write down makes so
much sense.

In my case, my plan was to fix what was causing my patients'
symptoms, so it never made much sense to me to mask symptoms
and not fix what was causing them. This chapter will detail which
therapies to use to fix the actual cause, what they do, and how you
want to use them.

Before I get into that, let me tell you a quick story about an elderly lady, Marge, who came to see me about seven years ago. Marge had attended a seminar I was teaching on stenosis, which is the narrowing of the spine. She wanted to know if I could help her, as no one else had been able to do so.

Marge was in her early eighties and could barely walk when she came into my office. She couldn't stand up straight. She was bent to the side and forward, and she needed assistance from both her husband and her walker, but even with that, she couldn't go more than a few steps without taking a break to recuperate from the pain and difficulty each step caused her.

She shared with me that she had never had back pain until about ten years earlier. As is the case with so many people, she did nothing about it for several years because it wasn't yet severe. She could make it through the day with rest and over-the-counter medications. But after about five years, she couldn't take the pain anymore and decided to see her doctor. For the next five years, she went from doctor to doctor for different opinions, resulting in prescription after prescription and injection after injection. Lots of doctors, lots of opinions, lots of medications, but no results. In fact, her condition only worsened.

Over those five years, she also had stints with physical therapy and, in her words, even "tried" going to a chiropractor. The pain had gone from basic low back pain to pain that radiated down both legs and into her feet, resulting in neuropathy.

While talking with her, I asked why she came to the seminar. The last doctor she had been to, she said, was a surgeon. He told her that she needed surgery, but he didn't recommend it because she was "too old." I felt bad for her because I knew her condition was extreme, but I also didn't know if I would treat her, since we have a rule of thumb in our offices: if we don't think we can help get a patient at least 70 percent better, then we won't accept their case. We have a very high standard because of the kind of work we specialize in. However, we have a success rate of about 90 percent with the most severe cases that we do accept because of that rule.

I asked Marge two questions: (1) What is it you can no longer do because of the pain that if the pain were 70 percent less you would be able to do? and (2) What are your goals and what do you want to get out of this? She looked at me and said, "Dr. Butler, I want to be able to cook for my husband again. I've always cooked for him, but the pain has gotten so severe over the last few years that I can't even stand at the stove. I have to sit. I also want to be able to go up and down stairs. I have a flight of stairs in my home, and I can't get up them any longer. And I want to be able to clean my house like I have all my life. I can't lift or bend from the pain, and I want to do that again." (Notice that her goal was to be able to function again, not just to get out of pain.)

I told Marge that we would do a very targeted exam and some testing, and that the results of those tests would tell me if I could accept her case.

The next time I saw Marge, I didn't have good news. Her spine had more damage than I had ever seen at that point in my career. She had severe scoliosis (curvature of the spine), severe arthritis, stenosis (narrowing of the vertebral canal), degenerative disc disease, and osteoporosis. The odds of her responding to our program, as successful as it is, were marginal at best.

When I showed her the extent of the damage, she was shocked. Most of the other doctors she saw never educated her about what she was dealing with, and she thanked me for taking the time to do so—even though that's part of our "over-delivering philosophy."

The toughest part, however, was explaining why we couldn't accept her case. See, the plan I'm about to go over is a plan to maximize tissue healing and functional improvement. The damage to her spine was so advanced that it was unlikely her body could overcome that. Keep in mind that if you plan to wait to get treatment, there is a point of no return, and Marge was at that point.

KEEP IN MIND THAT IF YOU PLAN TO WAIT TO GET TREATMENT, THERE IS A POINT OF NO RETURN, AND MARGE WAS AT THAT POINT.

She listened politely, and after she knew why I wasn't planning to accept her case, she asked me a question. "Why not try?" She went on to tell me that nobody else had been able to help her, and she didn't want to live the rest of her life in severe pain or in a wheelchair. She said that *any* improvement we could give her would be monumental compared to how she had been living, even if it was only 10 percent.

I thought about it carefully. I knew we could help her improve, just maybe not the 70 percent standard that we had. I also knew that when we were done, she would have "some" functional improvement, and that at the very least, it would stop the downward spiral and the advancement of her condition. So, I decided to help her.

Marge was introduced to the Butler Spine Program, the program I created that I believe to be the most advanced nonsurgical solution to low back pain. Before I describe each treatment, let me share with you the rest of Marge's story and how having a plan to follow is paramount to seeing the results.

First, due to the extent of the damage—not due to her age, by the way—I could tell that the condition in her spine hadn't started ten years earlier, like she thought it had, but closer to fifty years earlier! That means she had about forty years of painless degeneration of the joints, discs, muscles, and bones before she even had a symptom, and another ten years of progressing symptoms after that.

So, let me ask you this: If it took forty to fifty years for your body to develop a condition that was causing you pain, do you think you should feel better in four weeks? Probably not. As a result, I told Marge that we would need to work with her for about eight weeks before she would see any real changes beginning, and about twelve to sixteen weeks before she would see significant improvement. Keep in mind that she almost couldn't walk and that she had the most advanced degeneration I had seen at that point in my career.

Doctor's Note

After twenty-plus years in practice, my opinion is that most people who seek manual therapies for help, be it chiropractic or physical therapy, are grossly undertreated. They usually receive treatment based on something other than what it would take to correct their problem, such as insurance benefits or the provider thinking the patient will only accept a quick-fix style treatment plan. As a result, they never truly get better. If you value your future health, ask the doctor what it would take to fix it and not just to feel better.

We worked with Marge three times a week for one to two hours per treatment. (More on this later when I cover treatments.) After four weeks, Marge felt no better at all. She was a 10 out of 10 on a pain scale when she started, and on her twelfth visit, she was still a 10 out of 10. Most patients would have quit by then, but we told Marge what to expect, and she knew not to expect much. It was just too soon.

So, we continued for another two weeks, and she still felt no better. Boy, you must be frustrated imagining you're Marge right about now. But guess who wasn't frustrated? Marge. Because she had a plan.

Two more weeks went by, and guess how Marge felt at that point? If you said 50 percent better, you would be right. In fact, that week she came in and wasn't using her walker so much. She was standing up straighter and could walk down the hall without stopping to lean against the wall.

As we continued to treat her, she continued to heal. In the end, it took us just about sixteen weeks, and when we were done, Marge stood up straight. In fact, since she was standing up so straight, she thought she had grown taller. Amazingly, she told me she didn't need her cane at all anymore, but she still carried it because of the habit of having one for so many years. She walked the full length of the office without pain.

Most importantly, she was cooking for her husband, walking the stairs in her home, and keeping her home clean, all the things she wanted so badly.

How did we do it? Here's how.

Remember how I discussed that to help a patient get better, you had to know where the pain was coming from? I explained what makes up the spine and which tissues did what, and then discussed setting and achieving goals. Lastly, I told you that most of you, in my experience, get undertreated, meaning you aren't getting the correct therapy, you aren't getting all the therapy, and you aren't getting it for enough time to produce a result.

THE 80/20 RULE

So, I am a believer in the 80/20 rule. Roughly, the 80/20 rule states that 80 percent of your results come from 20 percent of what you do.

In this case, the timeline diagram I created for you is a rule of thumb that works 80 percent of the time. For the other 20 percent, it's up to the doctor to customize the treatment plan a little more.

In general, as you look at the diagram, there is a direct relationship between time/age and the severity of the problem. There is also a direct correlation between how many therapies you will need and how long you will need to get them before you feel better. (The moral of the story? Start early.)

Please notice that where you are along this timeline is not based on something subjective like your symptoms, but primarily on the examination and the test results—including X-rays, MRIs, and other tests—as the key data points, and the symptoms as a secondary data point. Also keep in mind that you only get symptoms after there is already too much damage to a specific area, and symptoms are the very first thing that will leave you, well before the real problem is fixed. So, symptoms are very unreliable; they are just a clue. You need objective tests such as X-rays.

STAGES OF DEGENERATION

1 1-20 YEARS OLD
REQUIRES 4-8 WEEKS OF CARE
CHIROPRACTIC
NEUROMUSCULAR RE-EDUCATION

2 21-40 YEARS OLD
REQUIRES 8-12 WEEKS OF CARE
CHIROPRACTIC
NEUROMUSCULAR REEDUCATION
PHYSICAL THERAPY
ACUPUNCTURE

3 41-60 YEARS OLD
REQUIRES 8-12 WEEKS OF CARE
CHIROPRACTIC
NEUROMUSCULAR RE-EDUCATION
PHYSICAL THERAPY   LASER THERAPY
ACUPUNCTURE   DECOMPRESSION
MASSAGE

4 60+ YEARS OLD
REQUIRES 12+ WEEKS OF CARE
CHIROPRACTIC
NEUROMUSCULAR RE-EDUCATION
PHYSICAL THERAPY   LASER THERAPY
ACUPUNCTURE   DECOMPRESSION
MASSAGE

When you look at the chart above, you are looking at the progression of spinal degeneration. What you need to get better is dictated by where you are in this chart. It typically takes years or decades to move down one phase of degeneration. In the discussion ahead, I am going to refer primarily to Phase 2, because that is when most adults start getting to a point where the pain becomes a chronic issue.

Prior to Phase 2, most people have symptoms that come and go, and therefore they don't take the problem seriously. In my experience, as people approach Phase 2, the pain and effects become more constant or chronic, and many are compelled to do something.

Doctor's Note

Do not approach your care with preconceived notions or biases. All these treatments work for their intended purposes. They have either stood the test of time or are supported by medical research. If you are biased or allow someone else to make you biased, you should not expect to get better.

RECOMMENDED THERAPIES

The following is a list of different therapies used in our offices and a brief description of the benefits of each. Keep in mind what I told you in a previous chapter, that every patient with back or neck pain has a *combination* of problems that is causing their pain. It is very rare that just one thing needs to be treated, unless it is in a child or young adult.

Before I get into the therapies, a disturbing trend I have seen over the last ten to fifteen years is that by the time someone reaches their mid-teens, they already have developed multiple problems in their back—primarily due to the advances in technology, such as cellphones, computers, and video games. These have resulted in more and more children living a sedentary lifestyle, causing problems that in the past wouldn't be seen until people reached their mid-twenties.

As a result, what we used to see in twenty- and thirty-year-olds we are now seeing in children and teens. Problems we wouldn't see until someone was in their fifties are now happening in their thirties, and so on. What's causing severe back and neck problems is worsening, and the effects are starting earlier. So, we need more therapies to help someone today than we did twenty years ago. The idea of a "simple back problem" has gone the way of the home telephone with the long cord, or the VHS tape. It's just rarely seen anymore.

Now let's move on to the therapies.

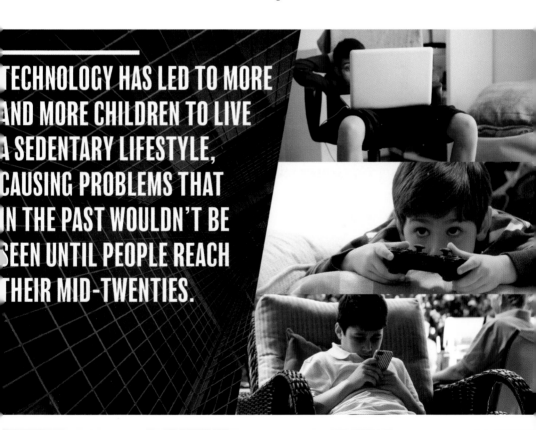

TECHNOLOGY HAS LED TO MORE AND MORE CHILDREN TO LIVE A SEDENTARY LIFESTYLE, CAUSING PROBLEMS THAT IN THE PAST WOULDN'T BE SEEN UNTIL PEOPLE REACH THEIR MID-TWENTIES.

CHIROPRACTIC CARE

Without question, chiropractic is the best way to solve the joint problems associated with almost all back and neck problems. A spinal adjustment is the safest and most effective way to mobilize the joints. With chiropractic, flexibility and range of motion of the affected segments is increased. Posture is improved, disc circulation improves, and nerves can function better. In terms of "bang for your buck," few things can help your back like the right chiropractor.

In addition to back pain, chiropractic's effect on your nerve function can help with a slew of other ailments (but that's another book).

NEUROMUSCULAR REEDUCATION

More advanced chiropractors utilize neuromuscular reeducation. There are two different types of muscles that control your spine: voluntary and involuntary. Voluntary muscles control global movements of your entire spine or region, movements such as bending and turning. You can voluntarily control these groups when you move. The involuntary group is responsible for controlling the position and movement of each individual vertebrae. These muscles are so important that you cannot control them voluntarily. Just like other vitally functioning parts of your body, such as your heart and immune system, involuntary muscles are controlled directly by your brain and central nervous system.

Neuromuscular reeducation uses specific exercises and movements to stimulate your brain to retrain these involuntary muscles and make a much better correction.

PHYSICAL THERAPY

Nobody does a better job of handling the muscle component of back pain than a doctor of physical therapy. Physical therapists' extensive training and schooling in rehabilitation is the key. For years, I have said that physical therapists and chiropractors are a match made in heaven for the very fact that the spine is controlled by joints and muscles.

Physical therapy helps increase range of motion, strengthens the spine against injury, improves posture and gait—the list goes on and on. Some people think about physical therapy only as it pertains to post-injury or post-surgical recovery, but I am here to tell you that it is also critical to longevity.

ACUPUNCTURE

Like chiropractic, acupuncture is a mystery to many people. Also, like chiropractic, its roots are deep in health and healing and not in back pain alone. It just so happens that more and more medical research is showing how incredibly effective it can be. Some studies show that it's more effective than pain medications, and unlike drugs, there are no real side effects. Plus, acupuncture produces actual results—it doesn't just mask the symptoms.

In our offices, we primarily use acupuncture to treat pain and inflammation early on, and to stimulate healing later. If you are "afraid" of needles, get over it. It almost never hurts, and even our most fearful patients fall in love with the results over time.

MASSAGE THERAPY

When most people think about massage therapy, they think about a spa or that it just feels good as a tension-relief strategy. That is only the tip of the iceberg. Massage therapy is a powerful healing tool. We have used massage therapy for many years. Massage helps to treat pain, inflammation, and spasm associated with back pain of all levels. In addition, a highly trained massage therapist aids in breaking down scar tissue, increasing blood flow to the affected area to accelerate healing while aiding the body in lymphatic drainage. The lymphatic system has a huge role in removing cellular debris and waste, which not only speeds up healing but has many other health benefits as well.

SPINAL DECOMPRESSION

This therapy has been a game changer in the treatment of patients with back pain who have degenerated, bulging, or herniated discs. It's the most advanced nonsurgical treatment for discs. The easiest way to describe it is that it is a very specific form of traction that opens and therefore decompresses the spinal segments in a specific area. It can be used for discs in the neck or in the lower back.

In spinal decompression therapy, the patient lies on a table and a harness secures one area of their body to the table. The affected area is put into a separate harness, which is attached to and controlled by a computer program pulley system. As a computer gauges the pressure needed to "distract" the spine, it gently stretches open the vertebrae. As it does this, it creates negative pressure in the disc, causing the bulging disc material to be pulled back into the disc and away from the nerves.

This description is an oversimplification but imagine holding a small water balloon in your hands and then squeezing it. As you continue to put pressure on the balloon, the water gets displaced and squeezed outward, eventually forming a bulge in the balloon out of the open end of your fist. That's what happens, in the simplest terms, to a disc over time or with an injury.

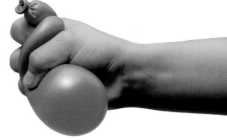

Now with the same picture in mind, imagine reversing the process by slowly releasing your fingers and taking the pressure off the balloon. As you do that, the pressure inside the balloon decreases and the part of the balloon that was bulging out of your fist decreases in size as the water moves back into the balloon. Of course, the whole process is not that simple, but you get the picture.

The success rate with spinal decompression is very high with our patients. In addition to treating the discs, decompression therapy can increase range of motion, flexibility, joint function, and muscle function in the treated area, all while reducing pain.

CLASS IV DEEP TISSUE LASER

Class IV laser has been as much of a game changer for pain, inflammation, and tissue repair as spinal decompression has been for disc damage. It's important to understand that lower level laser therapy such as Class III and below does not have the same healing benefits that Class IV has. Class III and below do not produce the same amount of power and cannot deliver the therapeutic effect as deeply as Class IV can.

Laser therapy is so effective that it is being used by professional and amateur sports teams all over the world to speed up the healing of sports injuries.

Laser therapy works on a biological level called "photobiomodulation," which essentially means that the laser stimulates damaged tissue cells to repair at an accelerated rate. Laser therapy also decreases pain and inflammation in the area it is applied to. Laser therapy can be used to treat patients with acute or chronic pain, and patients often report long-lasting pain relief.

What's so amazing about this revolutionary therapy is that with the high-powered laser, treatments are very fast. They feel great due to the soothing warmth that the laser creates, and there are no undesirable side effects.

PUTTING IT ALL TOGETHER

For you to successfully treat your back problem, you will need to know where you are in the timeline diagram from earlier in this chapter. You need to know which damaged tissues are involved and get the proper amount of treatment for enough time to allow them to heal. Only a properly trained doctor can tell which tissues are involved and determine which therapies you need from the list. There is no cookie-cutter approach here, so a proper examination and testing, including X-rays, MRIs, CT, and other tests, along with an interpretation of findings, are critical.

When I speak at seminars or to groups, I tell them the same thing I'm telling you now: Do not be deceived by outward appearances. It's easy to misinterpret the severity of someone's problems based on their age, physical presentation, apparent pain level, and so on. If you were to do that, in many cases you'd be wrong. The adage "never judge a book by its cover" certainly applies here, especially for doctors. Over the years, I have had patients in their sixties and seventies who had better structure and needed less treatment than people in their forties. I have had very difficult cases with patients in their twenties and thirties, as well. So, don't let age be the determining factor for how much care you need. In most cases the older a person gets, the more damage there is. But again, that's not always the case. And if you want to get better, you must do what your body needs to heal.

THE SECRET OF THE BUTLER SPINE PROGRAM

Remember Marge? Marge had one of the worst spines we had ever seen. To deal with cases where part of the spine is involved, regardless of age, I created the Butler Spine Program. I discovered something years ago that has been the secret to our incredible success with our patients. That is the simultaneous combination of therapies.

Most people with back pain that isn't getting better will tell you that, aside from prescription medications or over-the-counter medications, they have "tried other therapies," none of which worked for them. They'll tell you they tried physical therapy, or that they tried chiropractic, but what they didn't know, and what I taught you in this book, is that chiropractic and physical therapy work on different parts of the same problem.

So, if you are only seeing a chiropractor, they are the best at handling that part of the equation. If you are only seeing a physical therapist, they are the best for what physical therapy treats. The same goes for all the other therapies that I listed. They are the best for what they treat. The problem is that when you have potentially five or six things causing your pain and you're only handling one, you won't get better. In some cases, you might feel a little better while you're treating that part, but as soon as you stop, the pain begins to return.

Sound familiar? We hear it all the time. A patient comes to us and says they went to a chiropractor or physical therapist and that while they were there they saw improvement, but when they stopped, their pain returned. They would then conclude that "it didn't work," but it did work—for that part of the problem that they treated. Had they been treating all parts of their problem at the same time, they would have had a much better and longer-lasting response.

Many times, these types of patients will hop from provider to provider. Again, because they didn't get a complete recovery, or the pain returned, they concluded that the therapy didn't work, when in reality it was the *plan* that didn't work. They didn't have a plan to simultaneously treat all the parts of their back pain.

> **AGAIN, BECAUSE THEY DIDN'T GET A COMPLETE RECOVERY, OR THE PAIN RETURNED, THEY CONCLUDED THAT THE THERAPY DIDN'T WORK, WHEN IN REALITY IT WAS THE *PLAN* THAT DIDN'T WORK.**

So, think about it. They go to a chiropractor for six or eight weeks, and each time they go, they're doing the right thing for one part of the spine. They aren't treating all the parts, so the results aren't ideal. As a result, they quit chiropractic and go to physical therapy. Now they see a physical therapist for six to eight weeks, and again are treating one part of their problem, or one part of their pain.

The problem is that as soon as they stop going to the chiropractor, they start to lose the benefits of what the chiropractor was doing. They stop treating the joints and the motion segments, causing these problems to come back again. The physical therapist is working hard on the muscles, but if the cause of the muscle spasm and imbalance is the joints or the discs or the nerves, then the PT will get limited results.

The point is, if you're only treating one or two out of five problems, the pain will almost always return due to the untreated causes of the condition. You must treat all the problems that are causing your back pain, and you have to treat them all at the same time so that they heal at the same time.

And that's the secret of the Butler Spine Program. It is an intentional combination of the best therapies delivered at the same time and for a long enough period of time, to allow your body to heal all the causes simultaneously. So if the goal is lasting relief—if the goal is to live a longer, happier, healthier, pain-free life, which is our mission for you—then you must play by the rules. You must have a goal, know what's causing your pain, go to a facility that can treat all of those problems at the same time, have a plan, and execute the plan in full by allowing your body the amount of time it needs to heal.

There are no shortcuts, just good old-fashioned hard work, combining traditional therapies with modern technology and time. If you follow my guidance, then I believe that most of you reading this book will find the success you've been hoping for in as little as eight to twelve weeks.

- There is no such thing as a simple back problem anymore. Due to increased sedentary lifestyles among kids, back problems are happening earlier and earlier and are more advanced.

- Being younger doesn't mean you don't have a lot of problems. Only the proper testing and imaging can tell you where you are.

- Singular treatments rarely work. A properly designed plan should include multiple therapies for most people if the goal is to fix the problem. As you get older and your condition gets worse, you will need multiple therapies just to feel better.

- There are many safe and effective therapies with little or no side effects that will trigger your body to heal. If you don't treat all the causes of your pain, you shouldn't expect to get better.

- There is a direct correlation between how long you've had your problem (not how long you've had your symptoms), and how long it will take to get better.

- You have to choose where you go wisely. As we heard from so many patients, "I never knew you could do all of this in one place." That is by design—for you, our patients.

Visit drbradfordbutler.com for more information.

CHAPTER EIGHT

STOP BACK PAIN BEFORE IT STARTS

Care is an absolute, period. Prevention is the ideal.

~ Christopher Howson

*So many people spend their health gaining wealth, and
then have to spend their wealth to regain their health.*

~ A.J. Reb Materi

L et's be honest, very few people value prevention—of anything. If we did, as a country, we wouldn't have the world's most expensive health care system, we wouldn't have a massive divorce problem, and we wouldn't have so many people in poverty. My point is that we have a culture that mostly pays attention to important things after they're already gone. It's probably a bad idea to consider your marriage after your wife packs her bags or to consider your money after you've lost it all or put yourself in a massive financial hole. But that's what most people do. Instead of investing in the important things in life, people tend to shine a light on them after they have developed a significant problem. Then, to remedy that problem, people sometimes must go to extremes.

It's very clear in the American health care system that prevention is amazingly cheap compared to fixing a big health problem, but most people I meet see prevention as an expense and not as an investment. I always wonder about that. Further—and this is surprising—even after someone does lose their health, you would think that once they regain it, they would change their ways, feel grateful they dodged a bullet, and start living a life of investing in their health. You would think that, but you would be wrong.

I know of a surprising number of patients diagnosed with lung cancer who smoke after treatment and heart attack victims who undergo bypass surgeries that regress to the same lifestyle that created the problem. And dentistry is filled with patients who have extensive dental work, yet never floss or go back for regular cleanings.

Yes, it's confusing, but it's not surprising. Recently, I had a conversation with some dentists during a meeting with our consultant, and I told them that I think part of the reason patients don't follow instructions for prevention—for dental work or for their spine—is

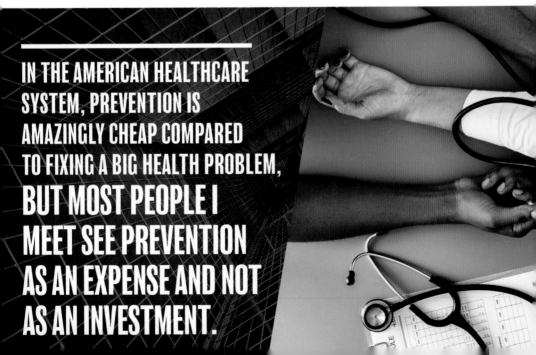

IN THE AMERICAN HEALTHCARE SYSTEM, PREVENTION IS AMAZINGLY CHEAP COMPARED TO FIXING A BIG HEALTH PROBLEM, BUT MOST PEOPLE I MEET SEE PREVENTION AS AN EXPENSE AND NOT AS AN INVESTMENT.

that all people hear about are new technologies and new treatments as they come out. As Americans, we have this false belief that if or when we do have a problem, there will be something there to bail us out. Unfortunately, that's just not the case.

I believe this is partially to do with that "bail out" mindset. In fact, when I meet with a new patient, I often tell them that it's unfortunate that we have to do corrective care, because chiropractic care and physical therapy, as well as massage and acupuncture, are all designed to prevent problems. However, when they have done so much damage to their body, we must use those tools in a different way to fix the problems. That means we have to use more of them more frequently and over a longer period of time than if they were used properly to begin with.

Let's use weight loss as an example. It's clear that if you eat a reasonable diet in reasonable portion sizes and get a moderate amount of activity each day, you will look and feel great your entire life. Europeans are a great example of this. If you live a typical European life, you eat smaller portions of whatever you want. There's no dieting necessarily, just less quantity. Also, in Europe they naturally move around a lot more than in the United States. They don't have to go to the gym two hours a day to stay lean. They just happen to walk more and sit less than we do.

However, in America, our diet is all over the place. We eat large portions (much of which is processed foods), we eat more often, and we move a lot less. As a result, we either go to the gym three to five times a week to burn it off or we get heavy. Now, once you're heavy, it's much, much harder to be lean again. Why? Because we waited and now we have to fix the problem. To fix it, we must go on what everyone knows as a "diet," which is basically deprivation. We must do it for weeks, months, or years, and we are miserable doing it. Many people quit because the symptoms of the deprivation are harder than just being fat.

Eventually, a weight problem becomes obesity, which results in other health problems that we have to take drugs for, many with side effects. Finally, when nothing works, the solution is to undergo a surgery where parts of the digestive system are cut out to force us to stop eating as much. Wow, that's a lot, right? Wouldn't it have been much easier to have eaten in moderation and moved around a little bit more, like our European cousins? And that's not to mention those who do stick to a diet and lose the weight, only to go back to the same lifestyle and gain it all back.

This entire example reminds me of the patients we meet who accumulated damage to their spine for years instead of just doing some basic things to prevent it in the first place, or at least slow it down. And even when we do an amazing job to help someone heal, feel great, and regain their function, most never follow our recommendations for maintenance care and home stretching, so they end up coming back again and again, and we have to do it over.

So here are some considerations for preventing back pain.

First, you can't maintain something that is already broken, meaning you can't come to us after twenty or thirty years and expect a quick fix. If you are a train wreck when you come in, we have to fix the problem first. Once the problem is fixed, then we can talk about maintaining and preventing.

Second, maintenance care is always cheaper, faster, and longer lasting than looking for a quick fix. Doing some or all of the treatments on a regular basis will give you the best chance at preventing back problems initially or keeping them from recurring once you have them treated.

Last, our body is designed to move. It's engineered that way. Therefore, if you want to think about it logically, the less you move, the more prevention it will take to keep you healthy and pain-free.

DR. BUTLER'S PRESCRIPTION FOR PREVENTION

Stretching and flexibility.

Almost all spinal problems initially begin with a loss of flexibility. Our bodies, and spines in particular, are designed for movement. The less flexible we are, the more stress the back is under; therefore, the more likely you are to have injury and breakdown.

> **Walking.** I am an advocate of naturally occurring ways to stay flexible, such as regular walking, which can be enhanced by not walking just on flat surfaces like treadmills, roads, or tracks. When you can walk on uneven terrain that changes elevation, it's even better, because it forces your body to move in different ways. Your spine, pelvis, and hips have to move in bigger ranges, and this is much more beneficial.

> **Yoga.** I believe that everyone should benefit from having a yoga instructor. Yoga is a fantastic way to increase overall body flexibility, strength, and wellness. There are many forms of yoga, and all focus on flexibility and core stability. Over the years, I have had many instructors as patients (and they get back pain, too). And one thing they all had in common is they recovered quicker because of their flexibility and core strength. For years,

I have tossed around the idea of bringing yoga in-house for my patients, but I have yet to pull the trigger.

Chiropractic maintenance.

When it comes to "all things spine," having regular chiropractic care is the number one way to prevent back and neck problems. Chiropractic care is one of the safest and most effective treatments you can get.

In his article "10 Research Benefits to Chiropractic Adjustments," health care expert Dr. Josh Axe stated that "If you frequently deal with symptoms like joint pain, backaches, or headaches, but are yet to ever visit a chiropractor for help, then you may be missing out on an effective and natural treatment option." He went on to say, "Millions of people around the world have experienced the incredible benefits of chiropractic care, a holistic, noninvasive treatment approach that has been shown to treat dozens of conditions."[34]

VISIT DRBRADFORDBUTLER.COM FOR A LINK TO DR. AXE'S ARTICLE.

What is chiropractic? Surprisingly, many people aren't aware. The Association of Chiropractic Colleges says, "Chiropractic is a health care discipline that emphasizes the inherent recuperative power of the body to heal itself without the use of drugs or surgery." Because of this, dozens of conditions are documented to be treated by chiropractic adjustments. Dr. Axe mentions ten in his article: back pain, headaches, neck pain, scoliosis, ear infections in babies, arthritis,

---

34 "10 Researched Benefits of Chiropractic Adjustments," accessed October 14, 2017, https://draxe.com/10-researched-benefits-chiropractic-adjustments.

bowel irregularity, improved mental clarity, asthma, high blood pressure, healthy pregnancy, organ function, and surgery prevention.

The chiropractic adjustment mobilizes the joints of the individual's spinal segments. This does many things for your health, including restoring normal joint range of motion, which prevents degeneration, injury, and pain.

Regular exercise.

Regular and consistent exercise is key in preventing back pain. In addition to flexibility, strength is a key factor in avoiding injury. In our clinics, we work with patients who are referred to us by orthopedists and spinal surgeons. I know what you're thinking. Why would they send their patients to us if we are so against surgery? The answer is simple: We have the best therapists.

Over the last several years, the trend has been to send us patients for physical therapy to strengthen their backs before and after surgery. Why? They have found that patients recover faster and with fewer side effects to the surgery.

Now, while I believe that most patients can avoid surgery, I also believe that surgery is sometimes inevitable. My formal position is that if you have to have surgery, then you will need preventative care even more post-surgery. The reason is that surgery doesn't fix what was causing the problem to begin with. In many cases, it's a big Band-Aid.

Also, surgery typically weakens the integrity of the spine, and you are more likely to develop more problems later. Preventive care is excellent, even after surgery. Strengthening the spine really is the key.

Nutrition and weight loss.

This is obvious, right? Maintaining a healthy weight is important in preventing back pain. Simply stated, the heavier you are, the more physical stress is transferred to your spine, muscles, and joints. As a result, they have to work harder and will break down sooner. It's also the case that, on average, when a back pain patient who is also overweight presents in our office, they tend to recover more slowly.

Yes, there are overweight people who don't have pain, but remember, pain happens after the damage is already there, not before. Eventually, the extra baggage will take its toll.

In this chapter, remember, I'm talking about preventing back pain before it happens. If you want to lose weight, I am a big fan of Tim Ferriss's "Slow Carb Diet" in his book *The 4-Hour Body*. I have seen significant results in weight loss, and it's also a very healthy way to eat.

As far as supplements are concerned, here's my position: eating a healthy, natural diet and avoiding toxic and overprocessed foods can help prevent inflammation and toxicity, making the body more resilient and less likely to break down prematurely. Also, healthy, natural foods give your body the building blocks to heal and repair faster. If you choose to supplement, I just want you to remember that they call them "supplements" for a reason. It's because they're supposed to supplement a healthy diet.

Regular massage.

Massage is a very useful tool in preventing pain and injury. We offer memberships in our offices because I am such an advocate.

Massage therapists are experts in relaxing tense muscles or working out trigger points and breaking up scar tissue. By getting a massage regularly, you reduce the risk that these muscle dysfunctions will lead to injury. Massage also helps you deal with stress, which leads to tension. Plus, there are significant health benefits as "pleasant side effects" of massage.

Early detection.

One of the best ways to prevent significant back problems is to get the right diagnosis early on from a chiropractor. Far too many patients waste years listening to TV commercials and getting treatments that don't work. I tell patients all the time that if they see something on TV, it's for a reason. That reason is that the FDA has deemed it safe for a non-trained, non-expert layperson to apply at home without supervision. In other words, it won't do much to help you, and if you screw up it won't do too much to hurt you, either.

So, over the months and years that you try self-treating, the condition gets more serious and harder to treat. My advice to patients—and here comes another dental analogy—is to think about your spine like your teeth, where you needn't panic if you have a little tooth pain that goes away, but you make an appointment and get your dentist to check it out if you have even mild or moderate recurring pain. It will save you time, money, and regret later on.

With your back, see a chiropractor right away. Why a chiropractor? Because we are the most highly skilled doctors at keeping the spine healthy. We know what normal, healthy spines look like and how to test for even subtle abnormalities. Medical doctors are trained more on disease and treatment of disease. What's the difference? Over the years, I've had many patients who came to us for second opinions when their orthopedist or sports medicine doctor was just flat-out wrong.

In one case, a young teenager came in with her mom. She had a history of back pain on and off since she was younger. She had an injury during competitive cheering and went to see the family's primary care doctor. The doctor said there was nothing wrong and gave her prescription drugs for the pain.

When we evaluated her, the evidence was very clear: She had scoliosis, which, if not treated properly, would get much worse as she continued to grow. Even her mom looked at the X-rays and was confounded. Had she not gotten the proper early diagnosis by us, and instead just took drugs for pain, it is very likely she would have developed serious spine problems by the time she was in her thirties and would not have known why.

> **HAD SHE NOT GOTTEN THE PROPER EARLY DIAGNOSIS BY US, BUT INSTEAD JUST TOOK DRUGS FOR PAIN, IT IS VERY LIKELY SHE WOULD HAVE DEVELOPED SERIOUS SPINE PROBLEMS BY THE TIME SHE WAS IN HER THIRTIES AND WOULD NOT HAVE KNOWN WHY.**

Remember Jason, the healthy fifty-year-old lifetime runner (in Chapter Four) who was told by his orthopedist that he needed a double hip replacement? After we tested him and found out that the problem wasn't in his hips but in his pelvis and lower back, we put him on the Butler Spine Program. Within days, he was feeling better. Within a month, he was 100 percent pain-free. And within six weeks, he was running again without pain. I wonder how much pain and suffering we were able to save him from going through had he had the unnecessary double hip replacement.

In summary, early detection can save you in more ways than one.

Change your environment.

Let's be honest, we don't work in the same environment that we did forty years ago. And just like our waistlines, our backs and necks have paid the price. The cost to your back of all the sitting nowadays is very high—the sedentary work so many Americans are forced to do may be the single biggest cause of back problems. There are a few reasons, but I will stick to two.

First, as stated before in this book, your spine was designed to move. If you are sitting for a good part of your day, you are effectively doing the opposite of what keeps your spine healthy. Sitting accelerates the breakdown of all parts of the spine that can cause pain. In an article from the Huffington Post titled "Sitting Is the New Smoking: Ways a Sedentary Lifestyle Is Killing You," Dr. James Levine, director of the Mayo Clinic-Arizona State University Obesity Solutions Initiative, is quoted as saying, "Sitting is more dangerous than smoking, kills more people than HIV, and is more treacherous than parachuting. We are sitting ourselves to death."[35] Okay, a little extreme, but he's got a point. Everything is worse when we sit.

The second point I want to make is that sitting is basically the same thing as flexion (or bending forward at the waist) of the lumbar spine and pelvis. Research suggests that sitting is the worst position for your lower back. If you think about it, sitting is like standing up and bending over at the waist at 90 degrees—all day long in many cases. And it can be made worse by twisting. So, if you have a job where you sit and turn to the side or lean to the side, you are predisposing yourself to injuring your spine over time.

---

35   Diana Gerstacker, "Sitting Is the New Smoking: Ways a Sedentary Lifestyle Is Killing You," Huffington Post, blog, from *The Active Times*, September 29, 2014, accessed October 14, 2017, https://www.huffingtonpost.com/the-active-times/sitting-is-the-new-smokin_b_5890006.html.

Personally, I have chosen, as much as possible, not to sit. I use a Varidesk standing desk and a shock-absorbing mat under my feet. The Varidesk allows me to elevate my work surface so that I can stand, and the cushion of the mat takes stress off the hips, knees, and feet. No, it's not as good as moving around, but remember, we're talking about prevention here.

The case for kids and prevention.

As I stated previously, most chronic back problems begin years or decades before any symptoms appear. I would argue that just being a kid and doing what kids do is a major cause of future back problems. It is my belief as a father of four and a certified children's chiropractor that all kids would benefit immensely from regular care.

It's funny to me that patients already have a certain understanding of "prevention" in other areas of their kids' lives. They buy hormone- and antibiotic-free chicken and meats for them to eat, they sign them up for sports and recreation to get them off the couch, they take them for their preventive dental and medical appointments—but very few take their kids to the chiropractor until it's too late, if even then.

I have treated several hundred children in my time. I have been to hospitals to gently adjust babies. I have helped children with their ear infections, asthma, and allergies, all through treating the problems in their spine. And do you know what's interesting? They all love adjustments. Kids get it. In addition to fixing small problems early on so that they don't develop into serious problems later, kids love how it feels.

When a family comes to us for care, it is their young kids who fight to get on the table first. Can you say that about their other doctors? In an era where we bring kids to the dentist early on to prevent problems, parents need to wake up to the idea that a healthy spine in a child is one of the best gifts you can give them. Not only will it undo what all their sitting does in school and while using technology, it will also have a significant effect on their overall health and immunity.

So, the concept of prevention is really a wellness model for our lives. We eat right and in moderation, we exercise and move around. And we go to the chiropractor, the acupuncturist, the physical therapist, and the massage therapist.

There's a story I've heard many times: Back in the early centuries, hundreds of years ago, "doctors" of the time would travel from village to village. However, they wouldn't get paid to treat the sick like they do in our current health care system. No, instead, they would only get paid if all the people in the village were healthy. So, their focus was on *keeping* people healthy.

THEIR FOCUS WAS ON KEEPING PEOPLE HEALTHY. TODAY WE HAVE LOST THAT.

Today we have lost that. The focus is on treating the sick and the broken. The vast majority of our modern medical system focuses all its attention, facilities, and marketing dollars on promoting the treatments of sickness and disease. It's no wonder we've all been convinced to do nothing until we are already sick. And what a surprise, we are sicker and more broken than ever before. I guess it's working. Yeah, I guess it's working.

Wouldn't it be interesting if we had a wellness model that focuses on staying healthy? My father, Big Bill, used to tell me, "Everything happens in cycles." In all honesty, we were talking at the time about the terribly outdated clothes he wore, but you know what? He was right. Now it's cool to wear the same "vintage" clothes he was wearing decades ago.

When it comes to health, I wouldn't mind a little vintage thinking, going back to a simpler time when being healthy and feeling good was the focus, and your doctors got paid to keep you healthy, not to patch you up and send you on your way.

- "An ounce of prevention is worth a pound of cure" couldn't be truer, especially when it comes to your back.

- Prevention is a mindset. You probably already do it in other areas of your life. When it comes to your back, you just need some new thinking and new habits. Prevention is an investment, not an expense.

- If you sit around and wait for a problem with your back—the old "if it ain't broken, don't fix it" line of thinking—don't be surprised when it happens. There are too many things that you do every day that will eventually cause damage. Sitting, repetitive movements, postures, and microtraumas are all daily occurrences for most of us. Wellness will prevent that.

- Maintenance and prevention are always cheaper, easier, and longer lasting than trying to fix a problem after it's there.

- The best way to prevent back pain from happening or returning is to focus on things that keep the spine moving and flexible, such as, but not limited to, walking, yoga, chiropractic maintenance, exercise, avoiding weight gain, massage, and early detection.

- Kids need chiropractic, too. Believe it or not, some research suggests that most of us experience our first spinal trauma when being born. Taking your baby or young child to a chiropractor who specializes in children (like us) will give them a tremendous advantage with their health overall, but also in preventing future problems with their back.

Visit drbradfordbutler.com for more information.

- @dr_bbutler
- www.facebook.com/drbradfordbutler
- www.linkedin.com/in/dr-brad-butler

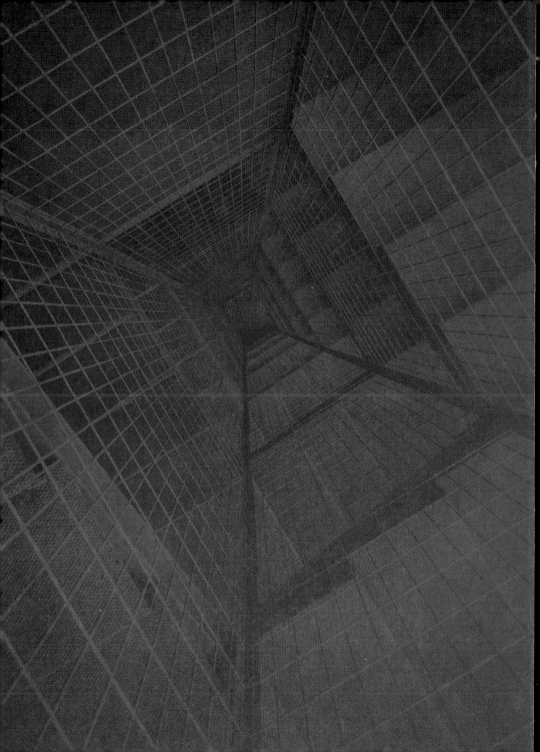

CHAPTER NINE

WHAT TO LOOK FOR IN A BACK PAIN PROVIDER

I remember how I felt when I received my diploma back in 1995. I did it! I was a doctor—the first doctor in the history of my entire family, including the Butlers on my dad's side and the Ribaudos on my mom's side.

On top of that, I was a chiropractor. I had a mission, and I was going to "change the world, one spine at a time," as my first business cards read on the bottom. My passion was to teach the world the power of the body to function at the highest level and how chiropractic was the answer to much, if not most, of the world's pain and suffering. It is not only a healing tool, but chiropractic will help you live a longer, healthier life, because it removes interference in the nervous system and allows the body to function at 100 percent and stay healthy so that you don't have pain and sickness.

Well, I did what I said I would do. Within two years of starting my practice, I was seeing over three hundred patients a week—on my way to seven hundred patients a week just a few years later. I was a hotshot in the profession, speaking at seminars, conventions, and professional gatherings. I was telling all my colleagues how I did it, and along the way I helped a lot of people. I changed their lives and those of their families. I helped thousands of patients heal from all sorts of things—high blood pressure, digestive disorders, asthma, migraines, ear infections (in babies), you name it. There is so much power in the human body, and adjustments help to restore it.

However, after eight years I realized that there was one group of patients who weren't responding to my care as well as I had hoped—the patients who came in with chronic neck and back pain. Yes, many did respond, but when they stopped coming in, the pain soon returned. And too many of them didn't respond at all or had minimal improvement. I couldn't figure out why.

Then one day, I was speaking with a friend, also a chiropractor, and he shared something with me. He was the son of a terrific chiropractor in New Jersey and had been treated his whole life by his father. Growing up, he never had pain, never got sick, and never needed drugs or medication.

However, while playing football in college, he sustained a severe knee injury. Years of degeneration later, he needed a very painful knee reconstruction. After the surgery, he was required to go for months of physical therapy, and while under care at a clinic, he noticed something. There were tons of people there with back pain, and the physical therapists thought PTs were the solution to the back pain, not chiropractors.

As we spoke further, I realized that when it comes to back pain, maybe we're both right and both wrong at the same time. My colleague opened my eyes to the fact that maybe it's not either/or, but "and," meaning that maybe we're both good at what we do and that by combining we can do even more. And that's how it all began.

After that, I went on a three-year quest to find all the things that were helping people with neck and back pain. I recognized that each "thing" that worked was good at treating something else that was contributing to back pain. Physical therapy, chiropractic, acupuncture, and massage therapy all played a role. In other words, the chiropractor helped by mobilizing the joints of the spine and taking pressure off the nerve. The physical therapist helped by increasing mobility of the spine and strengthening the muscles that supported the spine. The acupuncturist helped by reducing pain naturally and increasing blood flow to the area for repair. The massage therapist helped by decreasing muscle spasm and pain, decreasing inflammation, and stimulating blood flow for repair.

I also found new technology on my quest. I traveled the country and saw the doctor who was pioneering the use of Class IV laser to decrease pain and accelerate healing response and using spinal decompression to reduce bulging discs and increase mobility at the damaged levels.

After all my research and travels, I created the Butler Spine Program. In my opinion, it is the most advanced non-drug, nonsurgical solution for back and neck pain. We have evolved and taken back pain care to the next level. As a result, we are in the top 1 percent of providers in the country.

So, when it comes to choosing where you will go for treatment, ask yourself what you should be looking for in a back pain provider. Here is my list of qualities that I recommend to friends, family, anyone.

SERVICES OF MULTIPLE PROVIDERS

Look for an office that offers the services of multiple providers. There are a couple reasons for this.

First, when there is a team approach to patient care, the doctors meet and discuss each patient as they begin care. An office where doctors respect each other, value multiple opinions, and have different experiences can be invaluable to your successful outcome.

Second, it can help you avoid the "hammer and nail" syndrome that so many unhappy patients report to us in their past experiences at other clinics. (Don't forget—that was me years ago.) Basically, that syndrome states that to a hammer, everything is a nail. In health care, it's very common for a doctor of any discipline to think they are the solution to every problem. Unfortunately, they also have bills to pay. But when it comes to your health care, it's better to have options. So, when you call the office, ask what therapies that office offers to patients. It doesn't mean you need them all, but if you do, having them all under the same roof is crucial and convenient.

CONSIDERING THAT THE WORD "DOCTOR" IS DERIVED FROM THE LATIN WORD *DOCERE*, WHICH MEANS TO TEACH, I FEEL IT IS AN OBLIGATION OF DOCTORS TO TEACH THEIR PATIENTS.

PRIDE IN EDUCATION

Also, look for an office that prides itself on education, not just opinion. A shocking number of our patients thank us on the very first visit for taking the time to explain everything in detail, from what we are looking for to what is normal, from where they fit in to which therapies do what, and so on. Considering that the word "doctor" is derived from the Latin word *docere*, which means to teach, I feel it is an obligation of doctors to teach their patients. We take that very seriously at my practices, and I think it's wise to find an office where that is a priority. Asking questions such as "What is a typical visit like?" "What will I learn about the treatments?" "Will I know why I have a problem?" "Will I be taught preventive strategies?" are all excellent ways to determine if the office is a teaching office.

PATIENT-CENTRIC VERSUS DOCTOR-CENTRIC

Is the office what we call "patient-centric"? In other words, does the office completely cater to your needs when it comes to convenience, hours of operation, waiting times, payment methods, and so forth? If not, we call that kind of office "doctor-centric," where everything about the office screams: "It's all about the doctor."

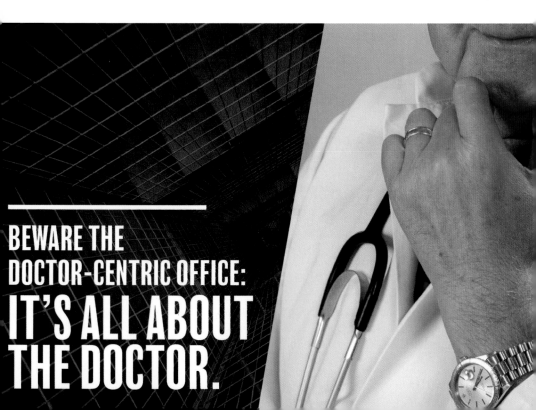

BEWARE THE
DOCTOR-CENTRIC OFFICE:
IT'S ALL ABOUT
THE DOCTOR.

Some signs and symptoms of a doctor-centric office are that it's difficult to make an appointment, either because you can't get through to them or because "their first available appointment" is too far off. When my mom was sick last year, we needed to get her an appointment right away. When my dad called, they told him that the soonest they could see her was three weeks away! He didn't know what I know, which is that's a lie. So, I called right back and let the woman who answered know that this is Dr. Brad Butler and my mother needed to be seen immediately, not in three weeks. Miraculously, she found an appointment; my mom was seen by the doctor the very next afternoon. The appointment maker said it was "professional courtesy." I call it a lie—the doctor intentionally pushes out appointments to make patients more desperate to get them so that they won't miss or cancel, fearing that they will have to wait another month to get in. This practice is common, and again, it's about the doctor and not the patient.

VISIT DRBRADFORDBUTLER.COM FOR MORE ON THE TYPICAL PATIENT EXPERIENCE.

Another sign of the doctor-centric office is purposely overbooking patients. Why do they do that? Because it's a business strategy taught by medical consultants and advisors. They call it "the overbooking method," and doctors use it to reduce the effect of no-shows on their bottom line. The consultants go on, however, to warn that using these methods creates patient numbers that are "often more than the clinic and staff can handle."[36]

---

36   Caroline Saint-Laurent, "Overbooking in Medical Clinics: Do or Don't?" PetalMD, December 23, 2015, accessed January 4, 2018, https://www.petalmd.com/blog/overbooking-in-medical-clinics.

The funny thing is that overbooking doesn't even decrease no-show rates, according to a Purdue report.[37] It increases no-show rates in the long run. So why do doctors still do it? Because they disregard the research and do whatever they want to do regardless.

In my experience, it's an insecurity thing. When a doctor sees an overbooked schedule, it makes the business side of their brain feel a lot better. I know of doctors in my area who triple- and even quadruple-book appointments. To me, that is the epitome of a doctor caring more about himself or herself than about you.

What about the staff? How do they look and act toward you? If you can't rate them highly, it tells you something. To me, the staff is 100 percent a reflection of the doctor's core values. If the office really cared about patients, then they would be friendly and welcoming and look for ways to make you feel good and respected. All too often, I see medical staff on their cell phones or gossiping about other staff—or worse, about other patients. To me, that says volumes about the doctor and what I can expect as a patient. Research shows that next to the doctor, their staff is the second-most important quality to a patient. If the doctor really cares, it will show in his team.

Some other doctor-centric symptoms to look for include payment options. This isn't the 1980s anymore, where most insurance companies covered everything and all anyone had to pay was a small copayment on each visit. Today we live in a different world, with high deductibles, high copayments, and limited coverage.

The doctor-centric office, of course, doesn't recognize that and demands payment in full. They want their money and they want

---

37 Bo Zeng, Hui Zhao, and Mark Lawley, "The Impact of Overbooking on Primary Care Patient No-show," *IIE Transactions on Healthcare Systems Engineering* 3, no. 3 (2013): 147–170, https://doi.org/10.1080/ 19488300.2013.820239

it now. There's no consideration for the fact that patients live on budgets and would benefit from paying for their care over time. As a result, many patients don't get the care that they need until it's urgent or an emergency and they have no other choice. To make matters worse, medical bills are one of the leading causes for a person declaring bankruptcy. That doesn't sound very patient friendly to me.

CLEAN, WELL-MAINTAINED ENVIRONMENT

Lastly, how attractive is the office that you go to? To me, that means a lot. It's a value thing, not a competency thing. If I walk into an outdated or rundown office, I think the doctor is pinching pennies and cutting corners. I could be totally wrong, but that's the impression I get. However, when I walk into a beautiful, clean, neat, well-maintained office, I feel different. Like I said before when discussing the staff, if the office looks unkempt and disorganized, it's probably because the doctor just doesn't care. If they don't care about their environment, I wonder what else they don't care about.

THERE IS A DIFFERENCE

These are the key things that I would want my family and friends to look for in choosing an office. There is a massive difference in your experience at a patient-centric office. In a patient-centric office, you will always be treated like a VIP. You will notice exceptionally friendly,

> **IN A PATIENT-CENTRIC OFFICE, YOU WILL ALWAYS BE TREATED LIKE A VIP.**

well-spoken, and caring staff in every single department you deal with. You will be seen on a day and at a time that works for you.

In our offices, we pride ourselves on having "the best

team in town." Our staff is exceptionally trained and excited to help our patients. We offer a same-day guarantee so you can be seen immediately and offer a "no waiting policy" that guarantees you'll never wait more than five minutes before seeing your doctor or therapist.

We also have a policy to never overbook. Unlike most other practices, this policy results in more time with patients, not less.

In a patient-centric office, education is a priority. A patient should be shown the respect of giving them as much information as they want, not as much as the doctor feels like sharing. Patients of ours regularly write our staff thank-you notes for being treated with that respect.

A patient-centric office looks for ways to make your care as convenient as possible. We offer our patients the convenience of having all the different providers they may need to help them under one roof. If we feel they need another opinion, we go out of our way to make an appointment on their behalf so that it is done in a timely manner. A patient-centric office recognizes that most people don't have an extra bank account where they've been stashing money for a rainy day when their back goes out, and therefore paying for care may be a challenge. In our offices, we offer multiple payment plans that allow our patients to handle payments in a way that works for them, not us.

Lastly, following research, a patient-centric office recognizes that today's patients expect an office that is modern, clean, and updated. It's no longer an option to get away with 1970s carpet and paneled walls. As a result, we make sure our offices are beautiful and functional, a place where you enjoy being. We regularly survey our patients about adding things like amenities that they want so that they have an exceptional experience each and every time they visit us.

It's a simple philosophy, really. If you see every part of the experience through the patient's eyes, provide the luxury of convenience, provide an exceptional experience in a modern facility, and surround all that with exceptional, caring people who are the best at what they do, the result is the happiest patients in the world. That is our philosophy at Oakland Spine & Physical Therapy. I encourage you to invest the time necessary to find a facility like ours near you.

TAKE IT ←·OR·→ LEAVE IT

- Possibly the most important choice you make in your quest to get better is the facility. Ask as many questions as you can. This is an investment. Choose wisely.

- Most offices you see are doctor-centric, which means that everything they do is done for the convenience of the doctor and the office, and not for the patient.

- For an exceptional experience and a better result, look for a patient-centric office. A patient-centric office looks at the experience through your eyes as the patient.

- Patient-centric offices have the following qualities: They provide appointment convenience by being open during hours that work for patients, same-day guarantee, and a no-waiting policy. They have incredibly friendly and knowledgeable staff. They have a focus on education. They offer the convenience of "everything under one roof." They have convenient payment plans. Finally, the offices are beautiful, modern, and constantly updated.

- Avoid doctor-centric offices whenever possible.

Visit drbradfordbutler.com for more information.

- @dr_bbutler
- www.facebook.com/drbradfordbutler
- www.linkedin.com/in/dr-brad-butler

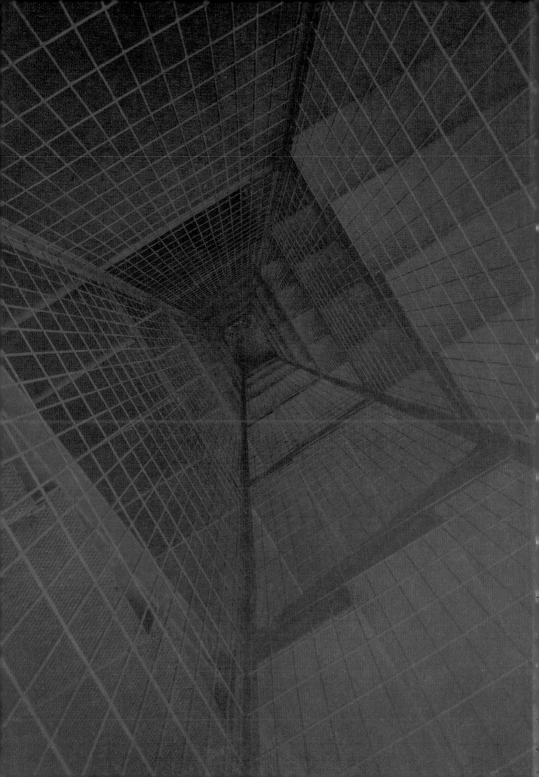

CONCLUSION & FINAL THOUGHTS

You are always one decision away from a totally different life.

~ Unknown.

Remember this: You are free to choose, but you are not free from the consequences of your choice.

~ Unknown.

My goal in writing this book was to give my readers straight truth, honest opinions, and a strategy to successfully negotiate the inevitable choices that most of you will face. I want you all to know that this book is intentionally written to be one-sided. I have chosen to do that to show you all "what's behind the curtain" when it comes to health care in general, but specifically back and neck pain. In doing so, I have painted an accurate, albeit controversial, picture of the truth that lies at the heart of all of this, and that is money—money that is being spent to convince you to think a certain way in the face of staggering evidence to the contrary.

Recently, I read an article that Phil Collins, the legendary singer-songwriter, was no longer able to play the drums during his "Not Dead Yet" concert tour because back surgeries had left him with a drop foot. I wonder if Phil and others who have suffered the consequences of surgery in the spine would have had a very different life if they had met me many years ago.

That's the real purpose of this book and the reason it comes across as edgy. Its purpose is not to tell you that your doctors are bad people, but just to say that they are trapped in a system and therefore must do what they have to do.

I often think about how easy it would be to convince the world that everyone should maintain a healthy spine for their entire lives if we had a trillion-dollar industry that would market that knowledge. Unfortunately, there's just not enough money in staying healthy, because there's no way to bring emotion into it. That kind of marketing money is reserved for things that they know people will be emotional about and scared about, such as sickness and death.

As a result, we have a drug industry and a government hospital complex that pushes the agenda of treating symptoms. They spend countless dollars in every media outlet possible to transform the way you think, and more importantly, the choices you make, so that they can get bigger and make more money without concern for the outcome.

Therefore, it's my job to rattle your cage and hopefully make you see things through a different lens. My hope is that this book, at the very least, can convince you not to follow the sheep to slaughter. Instead, I want you to ask questions. Questions will always be your best defense against making the wrong decisions.

Tony Robbins, the entrepreneur and life coach, says: "The quality of your life comes down to the quality of the questions you ask yourself and others daily." I believe there is a lot of power in what he said. I would like to add to it, though. I also believe that areas of our lives where we run into the most problems are those we don't ask questions about and don't look for solutions.

Those are the areas where we bury our heads in the sand and give up all our authority. Whether it's financial problems, marital problems, or—like in this book—health problems, they are the areas we develop serious problems in when we abdicate our responsibilities. Instead of asking, "What do I need to do to make this better?" and learning about solutions and actions, we ask, "What's wrong with me?" and get a simple opinion and accept it as true. When we do this, we give up our power.

My hope for you is that you have seen a completely different side now and you are compelled to take control, ask questions, and execute a strategy through your new knowledge base.

In wrapping up this book, here are some key summaries of the bullet points from my "Take It or Leave It" chapter summaries.

- As Americans, we are blessed with some of the best doctors in the world. However, our system is so corrupt and profit driven that you as the patient must question everything your doctors recommend. Your treatment must make sense to you.

- Because of our quick-fix culture, people are convinced to choose the most dangerous and invasive procedures first, even though they provide the worst results.

- Time can be your best friend or your worst enemy when it comes to treating your back pain. Untreated, the condition that's causing your back pain will always get worse with time, leading to physical and psychological damage. The results of this can lead to failed surgeries and opioid addictions, which ruin the lives of millions of people every year.

- It will never be easier or faster or cheaper to fix your back pain than it is today.

- You will have to think differently about your back if you want the results that you are looking for. No pill or surgery can ever heal you. They can only mask or treat the symptoms. Healing can only come from the natural processes of a properly functioning body. That is why people who have surgery often need more surgeries later on—because they never healed. It's also why so many people you know never actually get off pain medications. Is that what you want?

- Anybody can get better within reason if they do the right things often enough and long enough. Your body needs time to heal.

- Without a basic understanding of what makes up your spine, you won't be able to make the best decisions for your care. Be educated. Your treatment must make sense to you.

- Your back "is not one thing, it's composed of many things." There are six possible sources of your pain—joints, muscles, ligaments, discs, nerves, or inflammation of any of these. In most cases of chronic back pain, several of these are damaged, and therefore all of them need to be treated.

- Focusing just on the symptoms may not be appropriate or indicate where your pain is actually coming from.

- Research shows that more tests by your doctor doesn't equal better results.

- Your treatment goal should not be limited to just feeling better but should include a stated, functional goal. Without a specific functional goal, you lack a compass and your results will be limited.

- Caution: Don't just blindly follow "standards of care" that your doctor may recommend. Treatments have to make sense.

- Possibly the most important choice is where you choose to go. Choose wisely, because it matters.

- Beware of doctor-centric offices. Choose offices that are patient-centric. You deserve an amazing office with an amazing staff that fits into your life, not the doctor's life.

As the demand for this type of quality care continues to grow, maybe one day there will be an Oakland Spine near you.

We have a motto: "Exceptional care by exceptional people in an exceptional environment." While I would love to provide that for everyone across this country, there may not yet be an Oakland Spine & Physical Therapy near you. If you can't get to us, use our motto when you choose your office. If you start somewhere and you don't feel you are getting that, then don't be afraid to move.

Yours in health,

OUR SERVICES

At Oakland Spine & Physical Therapy, our end goal is to help people live longer, healthier, happier, pain-free lives. Our caring team is committed to relieving your pain and improving your life with a cutting-edge, holistic approach to health care. We do more than treat symptoms—we eliminate the cause of the problem.

Our services include state-of-the-art rehabilitation through:

- **Physical Therapy**

- **Chiropractic Care**

- **Massage Therapy**

- **Acupuncture**

- **The Butler Spine Program**

- **Deep Tissue Laser Therapy**

- **Spinal Decompression**

- … and more.

Each of our offices provide all services offered, so you can find everything you need to get healthy under one roof.

Services are provided by award-winning doctors and medical staff, ensuring you are always working with the best.

we offer same-day appointment policies (with a guarantee for emergencies) and free second opinions, and our no-wait policy guarantees that your care begins within five minutes of your appointment time.

Our programs involve no drugs, no surgery—just results—because we want you to feel great about feeling great again. Our goal is to have one hundred locations in ten years, and to be able to serve every state in the country.

Want to know more? Check us out at www.oaklandspinenj.com or reach out to us at one of our locations:

OAKLAND, NEW JERSEY
340 Ramapo Valley Road
201-651-9100

WAYNE, NEW JERSEY
1255 Hamburg Turnpike
201-651-9100

FAIRLAWN, NEW JERSEY
20-19 Fairlawn Avenue
201-651-9100

5